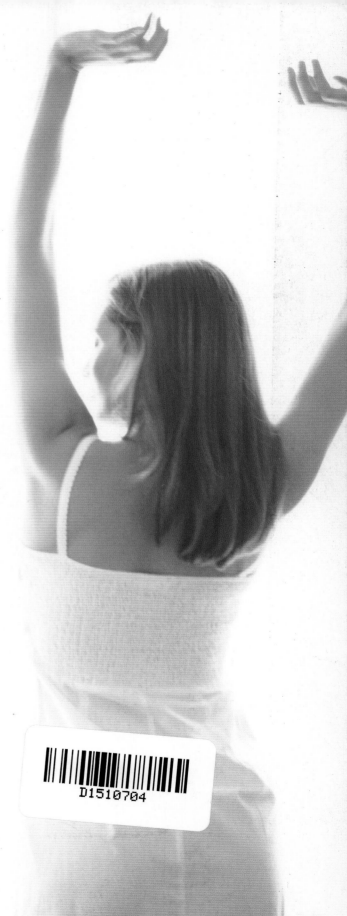

sleep
better
naturally

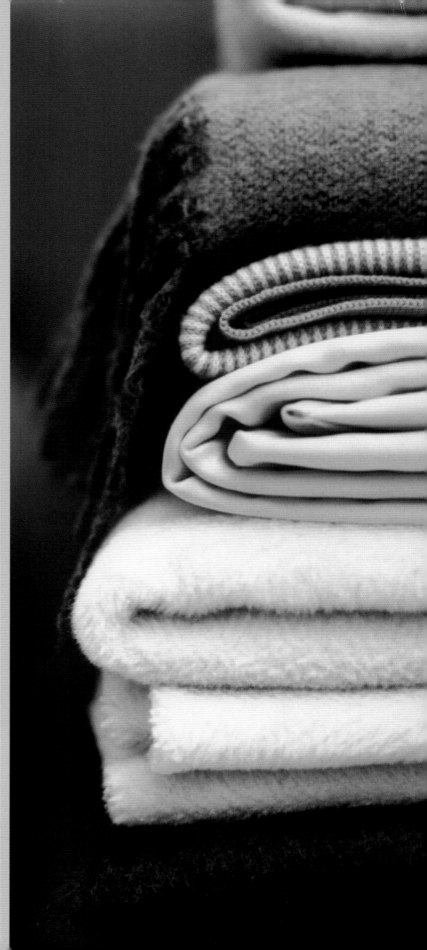

*To my grandparents, Charles and
Marie Fretter, and their home, where
I always slept soft and sound.*

THIS IS A CARLTON BOOK

Text and design copyright © 2006
Carlton Books Limited

First published in 2006 by
Carlton Books Limited
20 Mortimer Street
London W1T 3JW

Reprinted in 2008

A CIP catalogue record for this book
is available from the British Library.

ISBN: 978 1 84732 242 5

Printed and bound in Dubai

Senior Executive Editor: Lisa Dyer
Art Editor: Karin Fremer
Design: Barbara Zuñiga
Copy Editor: Lara Maiklem
Picture Editor: Sarah Edwards
Production: Caroline Alberti

The book reports information and
opinions that may be of general interest
to the reader. It is advisory only and
is not intended to serve as a medical
textbook or other procedural guide,
or as a substitute for consultation with
a physician in relation to any symptoms
that may require diagnosis and medical
attention. Neither the author nor the
publisher can accept responsibility for
any accident, injury or damage that
results from using the ideas, information
or advice offered in this book.

sleep better naturally

HOW TO BANISH INSOMNIA AND ACHIEVE A PERFECT NIGHT'S SLEEP

lisa helmanis

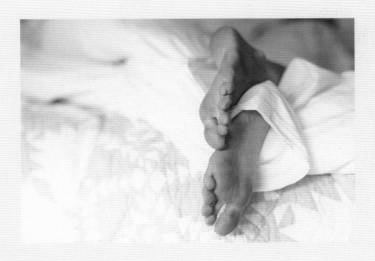

CARLTON
BOOKS

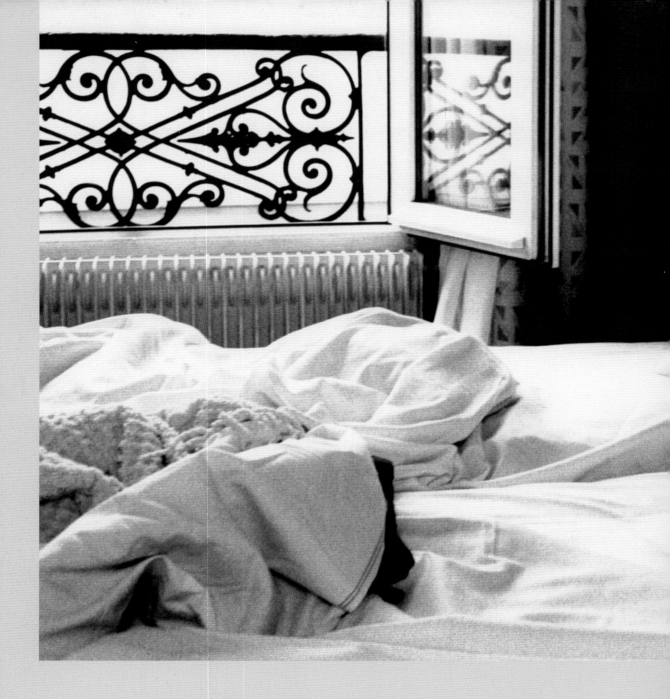

Contents

Introduction   6

1 Sleep Patterns & The Need for Sleep   10

2 Assessing Your Sleep Problems   22

3 Food, Drink & Sleep   42

4 Creating a Sleep Haven   58

5 Holistic Therapies   88

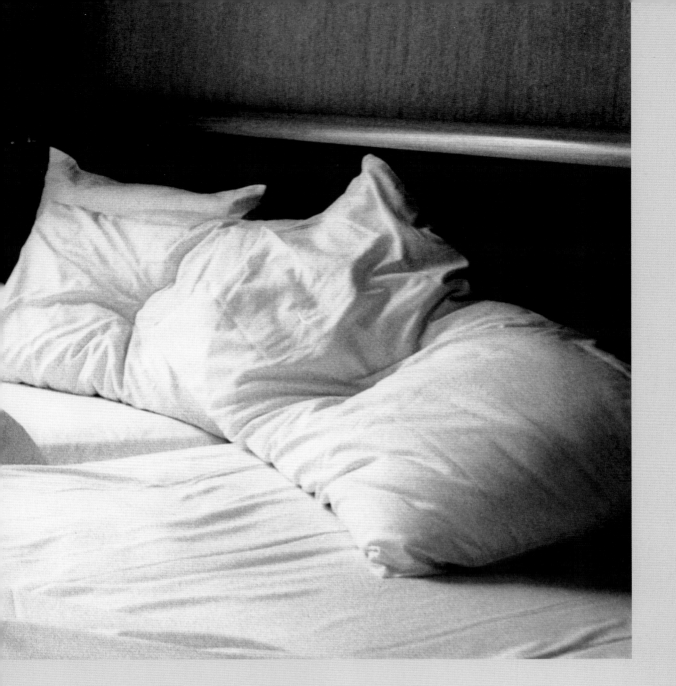

6 Fast-Track Strategies   **102**

7 Family Sleep Health   **124**

8 Sleep-Aid Programmes   **146**

Keeping a Sleep Journal   **154**
Reading & Resources   **156**
Index   **158**
Credits   **160**

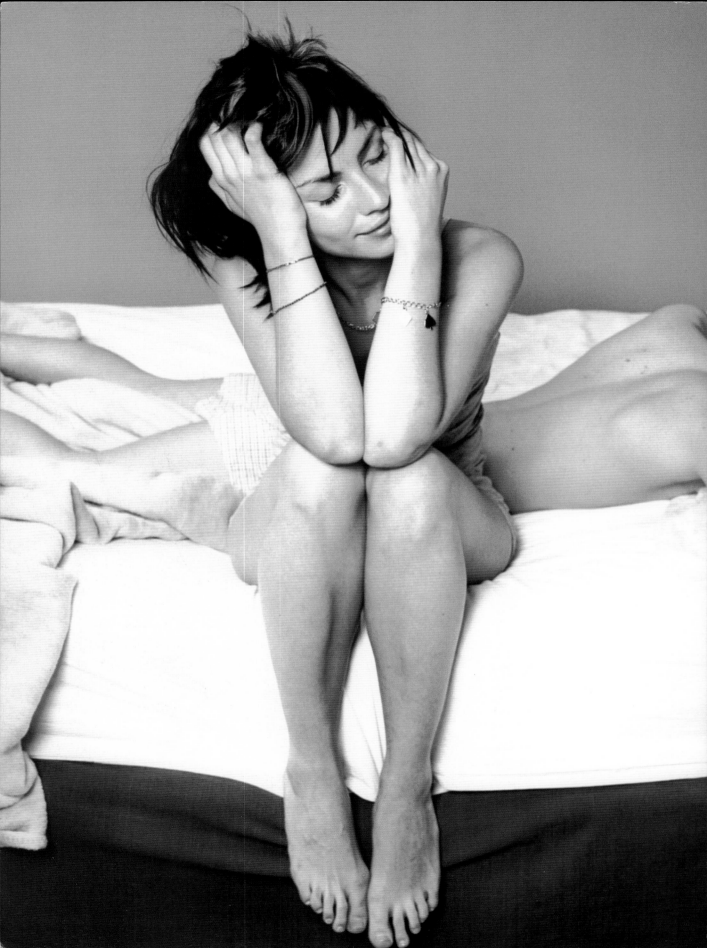

Introduction

OUR LIFESTYLES TODAY ARE ALL ABOUT being stimulated, entertained and excited. We regard the 24/7 culture that we have created in the Western world as an essential part of living and getting the most out of life.

Yet, while most of us acknowledge the importance of good nutrition and regular exercise in enabling us to take advantage of these pleasures, many forget the other essential ingredient for maintaining a modern lifestyle – sleep. Sleep is central to our sense of wellbeing and general health, but today's culture is increasingly marginalizing its importance and we are paying the price.

Despite the fact that we spend a third of our lives sleeping, research in this area is still relatively new. There is much debate on why we need it and the exact role it plays in our health, but all scientists agree that it is essential. Recent research at Columbia University in the USA has shown that little or poor-quality sleep can be linked to weight gain, with those who sleep only two to four hours a night 73 per cent more likely to be obese than an average seven-hour sleeper. This is in addition to the more well-documented effects such as mood swings, a predisposition to diabetes, irritability, poor concentration, anxiety, depression, reduced immunity to illness and memory loss. Add to this the immediate risk of accident and injury that fatigue causes (around 350 sleep-related deaths occur annually on roads in the UK, according to Awake, a body that advises the UK Department for Transport) as a result of somebody falling asleep at the wheel, and the scale of the problem becomes apparent.

LEFT **A good night's sleep can mean the difference between leaping out of bed with a satisfied smile, or reluctantly rolling over and pressing the snooze button, again.**

Even if you have never experienced extreme symptoms of sleep deprivation, you have probably suffered the misery of insufficient sleep at some time in your life. It is that unpleasant sensation of crawling from your bed, fuzzy-headed and disorientated, feeling emotional and frustrated, and more likely than not taking your unpleasant mood out on your nearest and dearest through the sheer inability to cope. Compare this feeling with the bright, positive glow you get from a well-rested comfortable night and it is clear why a good night's sleep is so important for tackling, and enjoying, the day's challenges.

Sleep is also important for learning. Tests by Robert Stickgold, a cognitive neuroscientist at Harvard Medical School, have shown that subjects who were allowed to sleep after learning new information or skills recalled them better when asked to repeat them. Those who had performed the same task later in the day with no sleep in between had poorer results. A lack of sleep quickly affects our ability to perform even simple tasks, articulate ourselves or control our emotions. It is also important in your body's fight against disease. When your body is fighting a viral infection, it will release chemicals into your system to make you lethargic and sleepy, thus giving it the chance to concentrate on fighting the infection.

Whether you believe sleep is a golden elixir or a nuisance that just makes the day shorter, its benefits can't be denied. It is important for your emotional life – depression, relationship breakdowns and inefficiency at work are all cited as results of, or exacerbated by, lack of sleep. It is also vital for good health, helping to prevent obesity, the onset of diabetes and the damaging effects of stress. Even your looks will benefit from a good night's sleep: beauty sleep is no myth, as any haggard new mother or father will gladly show you as they point out the bags under their eyes. Good sleep, in both quality and quantity, can dramatically improve your everyday lives and future happiness.

RIGHT Far from being a passive state, sleep can improve your mood, health, appearance, and even your relationships.

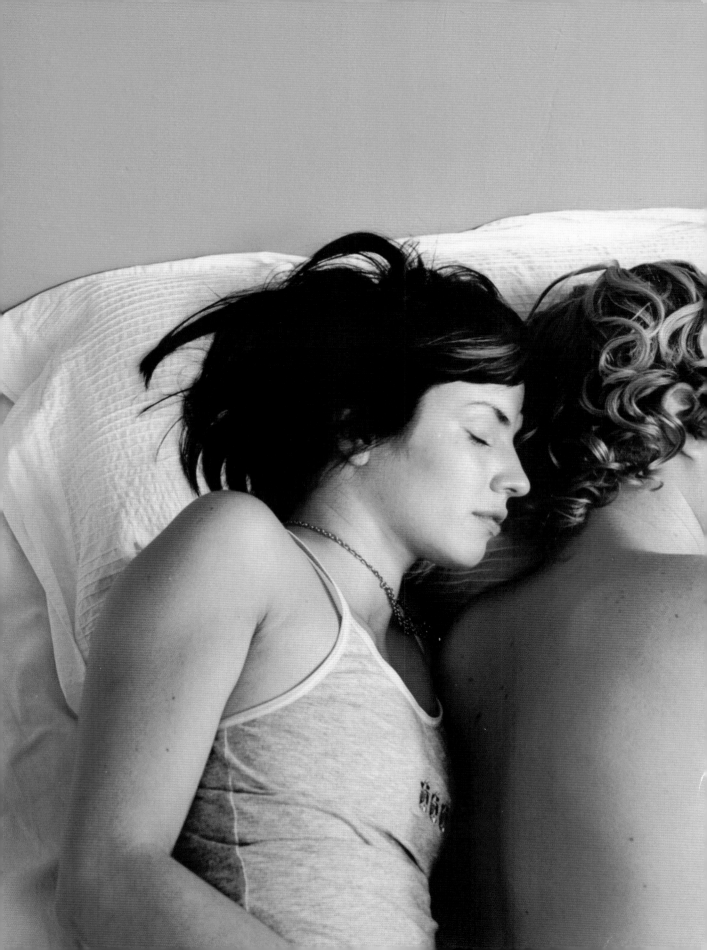

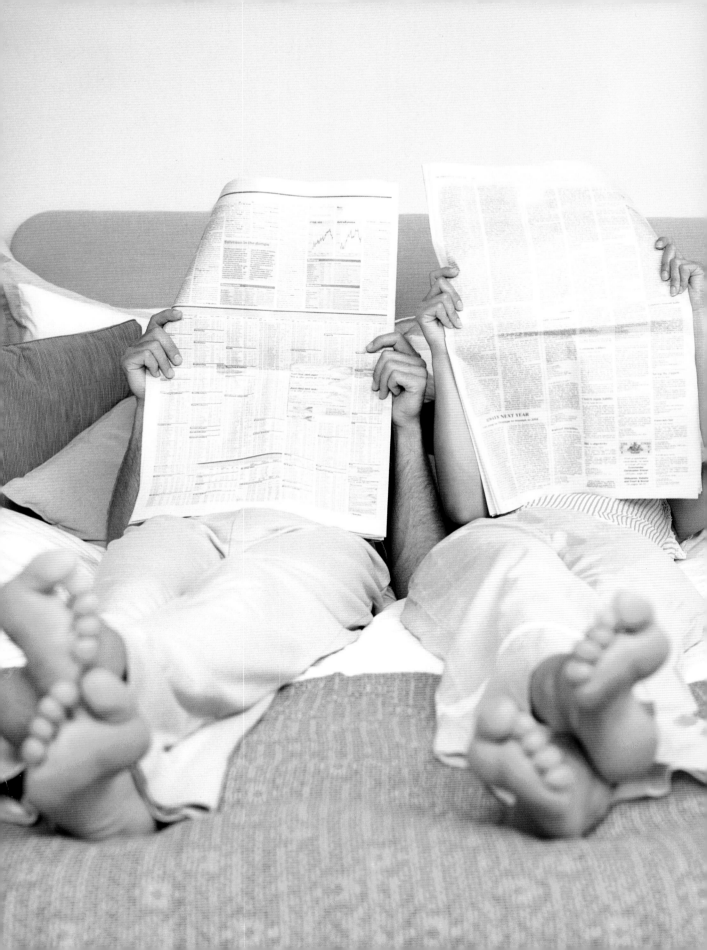

1 Sleep Patterns & The Need for Sleep

S O HOW DO YOU KNOW if you are getting enough sleep? Research from Britain and the USA has found that more than one in four adults feel they suffer three bad nights of sleep each week. On a very simple level, it does depend on how you feel – poor sleep will leave you feeling tired and sluggish the following day – though there are other tests you can do to see if you have a more serious sleep problem. First, let's look at a 'normal' day.

Our lives are governed by an internal 'clock' that sets out the rhythm of peaks and troughs we experience during the day. This clock is called the 'circadian rhythm' and it governs everything from hormone production to when we feel like going to bed. We are all at our most sleepy in the early hours of the morning and again in the early afternoon, which might be why work can seem like a chore just after lunch. The circadian rhythm doesn't work alone however; it works along with other factors, such as light – light can actually reset our clock, for example when we travel through time zones.

Through the release of the hormone melatonin, our internal clocks start gently telling our body, a few hours before we go to bed, that sleep is approaching. By releasing the stress hormone cortisol into our bloodstream, our internal clock also prepares us for the new day a few hours before the alarm sounds. For our body clock to get the

release of hormones correct, light is essential. This is why the glare from a streetlight invading your bedroom can make it hard to sleep – you might know it's night-time, but your body can't tell the difference between electricity and the sun.

So, if you feel perky in the morning, a little sluggish after lunch and then more alert in the evening, you are probably getting your sleep balance right. However, if you dread the sound of the alarm and spend the morning in a daze, tetchy and distressed, and you find yourself suffering from frequent colds and viruses, you are probably sleep-deprived. There can be a large number of reasons for this, such as:

• Birth of a new baby
• Menopause
• Pressure at work
• Overactive thyroid gland
• Post-traumatic Stress Disorder
• Anxiety
• Bereavement
• Illness
• Depression
• ME or Chronic Fatigue Syndrome

LEFT **Most of us do more than just sleep in bed. How we spend time in the bedroom also changes constantly throughout our lives.**

- Shift work
- Penchant for late-night parties
- Overuse of stimulants such as coffee, alcohol and nicotine
- Sleep apnoea (a breathing difficulty that causes you to wake repeatedly)
- Snoring partner
- Jet lag
- Delayed Sleep Phase Syndrome (DSPS), making it impossible to fall asleep until early morning
- Ageing.

It may even be the short-term, regular effects of another cycle; premenstrual syndrome (also known as premenstrual tension) is known to cause sleeplessness. Although chronic sleep deprivation (which means you are literally falling asleep during the day, and which can even be caused by missing a single night of sleep) can be rectified over a couple of nights, a slow buildup of sleep loss, even an hour or so a night, can affect your long-term health and make you susceptible to illness, weight gain and even premature death.

HOW SLEEP WORKS

While we are still unclear about the exact role of sleep, scientific research has revealed more about the form it takes. Sleep has two main states – REM (Rapid Eye Movement) and non-REM.

Within the non-REM stage there are four distinct stages. The first stage is very short, lasting about 10 minutes. It allows the muscles to relax and the brainwave patterns begin to slow down. During this stage you are very easy to wake, and as it begins, you may have that sensation of 'nodding off', with little rouses into consciousness.

To an observer, stage two looks very much like stage one, however an EEG (a graph called an electroencephalogram that depicts the pattern of brain waves produced by the brain) shows that there is a change in the type of brain waves being produced. A single wave, called K complexes, is followed by a sleep spindle (named after the spindle shape it makes on the EEG screen). It

would take a louder noise or firmer prod to rouse you from this stage, but you are still considered to be in the 'entering' stage of sleep.

About 10–15 minutes after the onset of stage two, you enter stage three. The brain waves are now slow and make rolling shapes on the EEG screen, indicating a very deep sleep. Your heart rate and blood pressure fall, your breathing is slow and regular, and you will need a ringing phone, shouting or shaking to bring you back to the waking world, which would find you groggy and disorientated and probably not very happy (which is also how you would feel if woken during stage four). This is followed by the last stage of non-REM sleep, which is even deeper. Your muscles are now totally relaxed and you are difficult to wake up – an onlooker might be tempted to use the phrase 'dead to the world'. It is during these deep stages that our body carries out its repair work, fights any illness or damage and, in men, releases the growth hormone. This is the sleep that truly refreshes us. As the night wears on, the deep stages of sleep become shorter and the REM stages lengthen.

These four non-REM stages described above take you approximately one hour into your first sleep cycle. You will then re-emerge towards consciousness and experience a brief awakening that you won't remember; this is often when you turn over or grab back some of the sheets. (Dr Paul Caldwell in his book *Sleep Really Well* suggests that this may be due to an evolutionary need to check one's environment for danger, as in deep sleep we are very vulnerable.) After this you start REM sleep, where high-frequency waves begin to appear on the EEG screen. Your brain has now started to create some alpha and beta waves, which are similar to the ones produced when we are awake. You are probably dreaming and your eyeballs are

RIGHT **The body has its own pacing mechanism – the circadian rhythm – that decides when we feel perky or sleepy; we can choose to respect it, or not.**

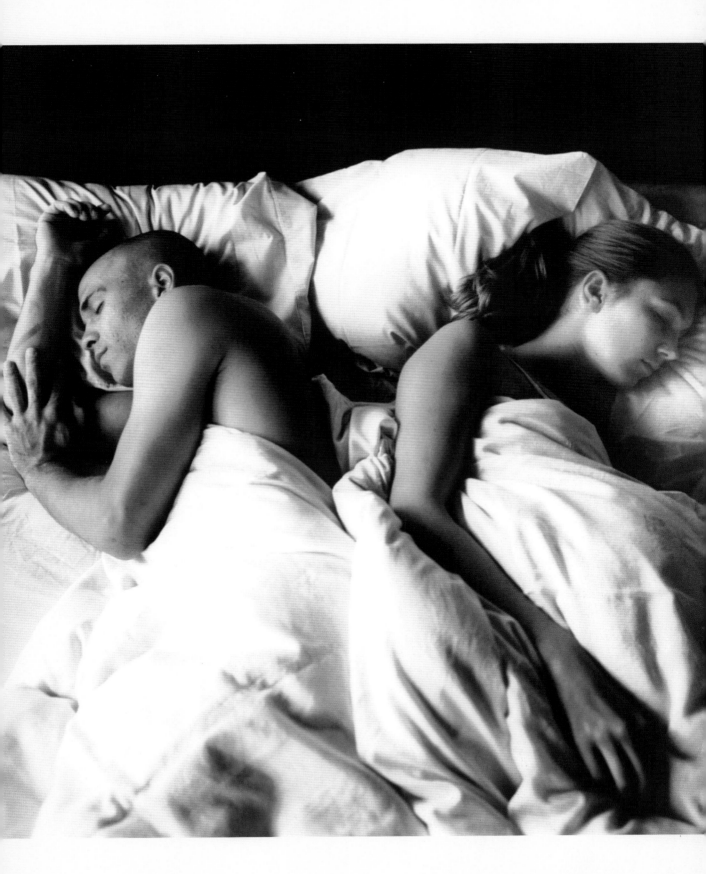

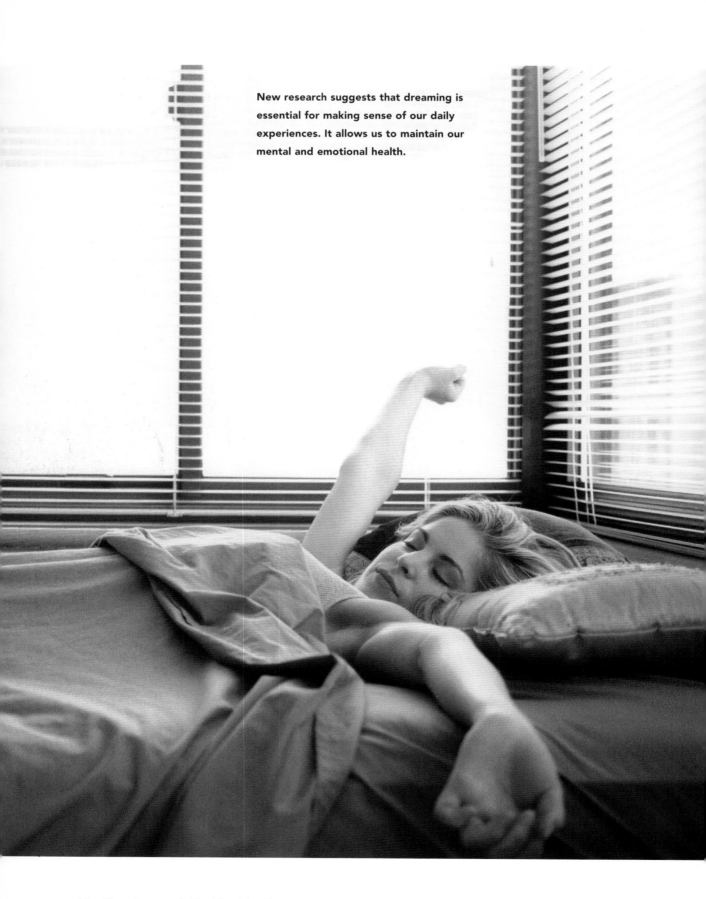

New research suggests that dreaming is essential for making sense of our daily experiences. It allows us to maintain our mental and emotional health.

moving under their lids, which is what gives REM sleep its name (you can also dream in non-REM sleep, but these dreams tend to be simple and short). Although dreams seem very real and physically active, your body won't act out your dreams as your muscles are paralyzed in this stage and you remain motionless (some scientists believe that this is the body's way of preventing you from harming yourself). Sleepwalking is likely to happen in the non-REM part of your sleep, which isn't accompanied by paralysis.

A full cycle of non-REM and REM sleep takes about 90 minutes: about 60 minutes in the various forms of non-REM sleep, and between 10 minutes and up to 30 minutes of REM, with the REM sleep periods lengthening gradually throughout the night. In total, 20 per cent of an average night will be spent dreaming. (Age also affects the proportion of sleep types you have, with less REM as you get older.) Once you have completed a full cycle, you return to the first, non-REM, stage and repeat it. The number of cycles you perform depends on how long you sleep, but most people wake up in the final cycle of REM sleep, which is why we often remember our dreams. As you are naturally closer to the waking state at this time, you will feel more refreshed emerging from this sleep stage.

Sleep watches have been developed, which monitor your body and look for these 'almost awake' moments, triggering your morning alarm clock and ensuring you wake during these parts of your cycle. Of course, getting the right amount of sleep would make this a natural occurrence, but for those who need to be up at certain times, setting a window of about 20 minutes for the watch to seek out the optimum, least distressing time to sound the alarm can make the interruption less agonizing.

RIGHT Restless sleep and rhythmic jerking of the feet or legs can be a sign of periodic limb movement in sleep (PLMS), a disorder that impairs sleep quality.

There can be a few unexpected additions to this sleep pattern. For instance, despite a conviction that we may have slept soundly throughout the whole night, we usually wake up from the shallower phases of sleep several times – we just don't remember doing it. Some research has shown that muscles in the body do not need sleep, just periods of rest. All research does agree that sleep is essential for the brain. Electroencephalogram (EEG) results show that the parts of the brain that deal with emotional issues, for example, are very active. This has fostered the new belief that we need sleep to process our daily feelings and consolidate our memories. Some scientists say we only dream the memories and situations that are meaningful to us, while others consider dreaming to be a way of shedding information that is surplus to requirements or trivial. Either way, it seems to be an essential part of our mental wellbeing.

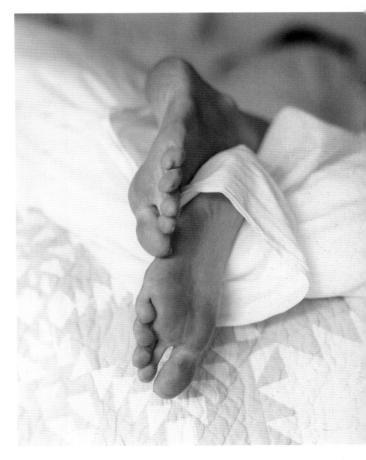

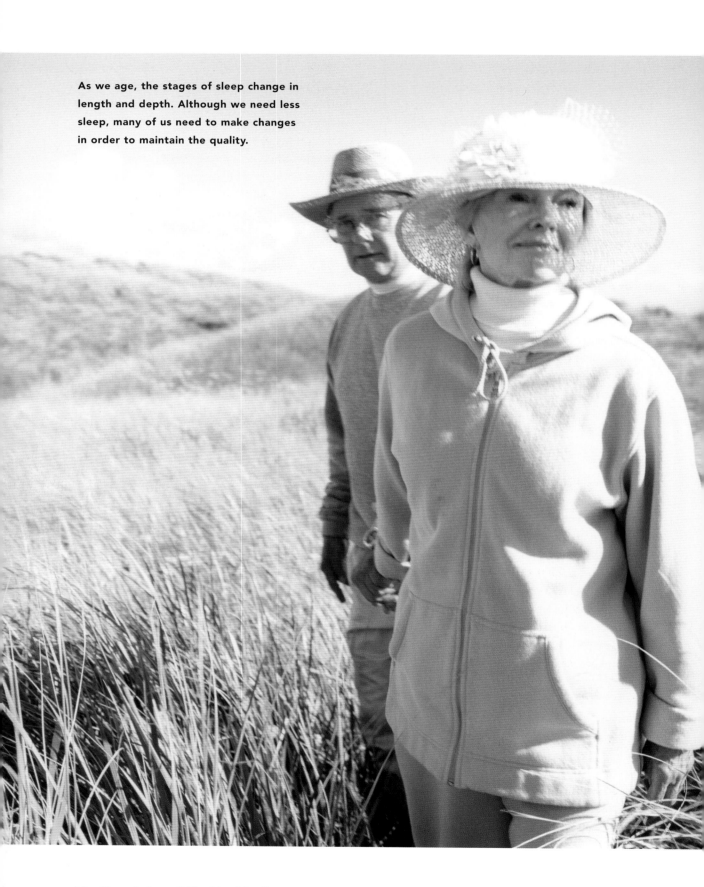

As we age, the stages of sleep change in length and depth. Although we need less sleep, many of us need to make changes in order to maintain the quality.

NATURAL EFFECTS ON YOUR SLEEP PATTERNS

There are two other factors that need to be considered when understanding your sleep patterns. Both are entirely natural and exert a profound influence on the way that we sleep.

Ageing

As well as the circadian rhythm (see page 11) and our lark or owl status (see below), we are ruled by the basic cycle of life. Ageing greatly influences our sleep patterns; six-month-old babies sleep for up to 16 hours a day, teenagers need about nine, adults need about eight, and from middle age the length and quality of sleep often gradually decreases. Older people report more instances of night-time awakenings, insomnia and unwanted early waking. They can often find sleep affected by illness or other problems, such as snoring and also have less REM sleep, but, due to more frequent night-time awakenings, they remember more dreams.

Larks and Owls

We are all either 'larks' (or 'early birds'), which means we prefer to rise early and go to bed early, or 'owls', which makes us prone to late nights and later rising times. This can change during our lifetime – most of us will remember being owls when we were teenagers! Your lifestyle pattern, such as taking children to school or shift work, may force you into a set regime, but your natural inclination will decide whether or not you will be at your best when you wake up. Larks are often breezy and perky in the mornings, but fade fast in the evenings. Owls, on the other hand, will loathe an early-morning start but find that they are full of energy at night. In an ideal world, we would start work at the time best suited to our disposition.

RIGHT **Understanding your own natural sleep disposition will help you to find a pattern that optimizes the effectiveness of both your waking and dreaming hours.**

SLEEP AND YOUR IMMUNE SYSTEM

In our hectic every day lives, it is easy to sacrifice sleep in order to meet the many demands of chaotic schedules. We need to realize, however, that in doing this we are depleting our natural resources that fight infection and help us to cope with daily demands. The immune system is our defence against illness and it filters out the damaged and defective body cells. A well-operating system can seek out a virus and minimize it to a snuffle, rather than create a sledgehammer that wipes us out for weeks. The lymph nodes produce the cells that attack invaders. They are located in your neck, armpits and groin, which is why they feel swollen when you are ill – it means they are doing their job properly. A healthy immune system needs vitamins and nutrients to maintain it, and most importantly it needs sleep. A lack of sleep suppresses your immune system and prevents it from being able to fight infection effectively.

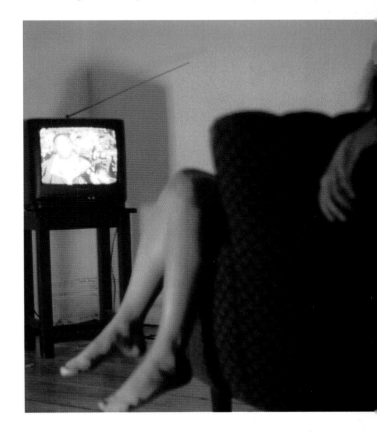

HOW MUCH SLEEP IS ENOUGH?

The standard figure that has been recommended by most healthcare professionals over the years is eight hours per night, although older people may need less sleep and children need a lot more, as they are growing. Everyone's needs vary, but research carried out at Stanford University, California, under the eye of William Dement, a highly respected expert in the field of sleep research, showed that most people had a sleep deficit of around 25–30 hours. Once people had recovered from their sleep deficit, they generally settled into a natural pattern of around eight hours a night, with women sleeping 20 minutes more a night than men. When you consider the fact that scientist Paul Martin (in his book *Counting Sheep*) estimated that most adults average 6.7 hours before a working day and 7.1 hours before a day off, you can see how easy it is to create a sleep deficit that leaves you yawning.

So how do you work out your needs? The time that it takes us to fall asleep from lying down to attempting sleep is called the Sleep Latency Period, and this can be used to measure how tired you are. You lie in a darkened room in the middle of the day, ready to take a nap. Everything is normal except that you have your arm hanging off the edge of the bed and with it you hold a spoon, over a metal tray, or something else that will make a clattering noise when the spoon is dropped. You write down the time you lay down and the time you are awoken by the clatter when the spoon slips out of your hand and onto the tray. If it takes you between 15 and 20 minutes, you are pretty normal; around ten minutes and you may have accumulated a sleep deficit; less than five minutes and you are suffering from a problematic lack of sleep.

If this method seems unscientific, try the Epworth Scale that has been developed by Murray Johns at the Sleep Disorders Unit, Epworth Hospital, Melbourne, Australia, and first published in 1991. Answer the questions in the box at the top of the page using the points system.

How likely are you to doze off in the following situations?

Never – 0

Occasionally – 2

Often – 3

Most of the time – 4

- **Sitting and reading**
- **Watching television**
- **Sitting in a public place, such as a theatre or at a meeting**
- **As a passenger in a car for an hour without a break**
- **Lying down in the afternoon**
- **Sitting talking to someone**
- **Sitting quietly after an alcohol-free lunch**
- **In a car, stopped for a few minutes in a traffic jam**

If you score more than ten, you are probably not getting enough sleep or getting poor-quality sleep.

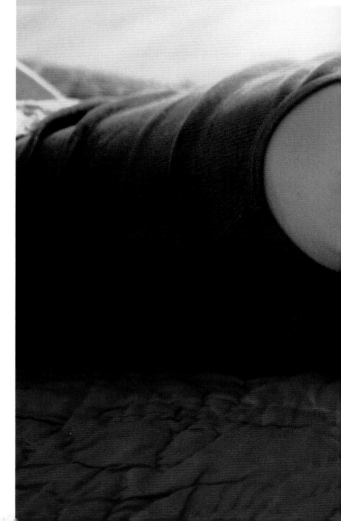

NAPPING – A QUICK RESTORATIVE

There was a time when only cats and grandparents could get away with napping, but as the restorative power of sleep becomes better understood, health professionals have now begun to advocate its advantages. Far from being the habit of a sloth, a well-timed nap can improve your state of mind and your energy levels. In many cultures, napping is an accepted and promoted way of living, the Spanish siesta being a prime example.

The optimum length for napping is still open to debate, but if you find that groggy feeling after a nap disruptive or unpleasant, limit your nap to between 10 and 20 minutes. For a proper break, nap for between 60 and 90 minutes. Everyone has slightly different needs, so experiment, but also make sure you don't overdo it. If you nap too much during the day, you won't sleep well at night, so you shouldn't be using napping in order to catch up on the sleep you missed by being awake the night before.

BELOW **Napping is no longer seen as a sign of laziness. A quick snooze can help boost your brain power and resilience, so curl up and doze.**

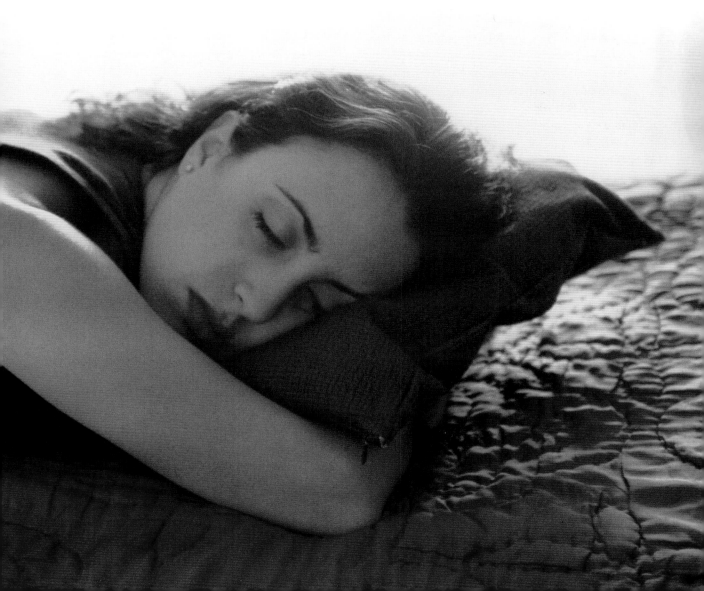

THE ROLE OF EXERCISE IN GOOD SLEEP

While most people would agree with the idea that physical exhaustion promotes sleep, it isn't, however, quite as simple as it would first seem. Studies have shown that muscles can remain healthy if given periods of rest, but that does not have to be sleep. The growth hormone repairs and maintains the body, and in men (not women) is mainly made during sleep. After exercise, the amount of slow wave sleep when this hormone is released is shown to increase – although some scientists argue that the change is modest.

So why do people feel that exercise so greatly improves their sleep if it is not wholly reflected in research? Well, exercise is wonderful for the body and our state of mind. Many conditions, from depression to premenstrual tension, are improved by taking exercise. As well as weight loss (which can help eliminate snoring), it can also reduce tension in our muscles, which can contribute to RSL (Restless Leg Syndrome, see page 31), and boost the brain chemical serotonin, which makes us feel good and pacifies all those little anxieties that can keep us awake. Repetitive physical activities, such as mountain walking or kayaking, also help the brain enter the alpha stage. This is when your conscious mind is focused on the activity, allowing it to connect with your subconscious mind, where solutions and ideas begin to make themselves apparent. This kind of activity may help you to solve that work crisis, which in turn will help you to then get better rest. Doing some physical exercise three times a week, even only 20 minutes at a time, will help your frame of mind and your physical frame.

GETTING BACK ON TRACK

Whatever the reason for losing your natural balance, there are many ways in which you can regain control. Losing sleep can often result in a nasty feeling of being overtired, and unable to sleep no matter how desperate you are. This situation can bring on insomnia (see page 24), a condition all the more frustrating in that worrying about it seems only to exacerbate it. Feeling tired magnifies the helpless feeling that accompanies insomnia – spotting a pattern yet?

The great news is that, far from being helpless, there are many ways in which you can improve the quality of your slumber. In the following chapters we will look at some of these ways, such as techniques to combat negative stress and lifestyle pressures, how to eliminate aggravating dietary factors and integrate sleep-friendly foods, and how to create a sleep-inducing haven, including pleasurable pre-sleep rituals. In addition, all-natural alternative and holistic therapies and re-training techniques can replace or supplement orthodox medicine.

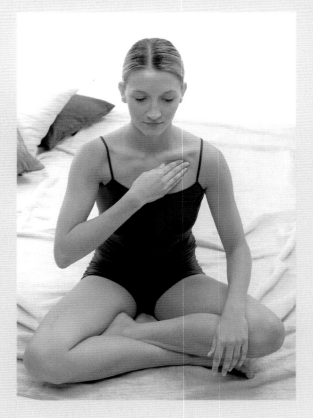

LEFT AND OPPOSITE **Seeking out ways to relieve stress and worry – such as yoga, self-massage or simply indulging in peaceful bedtime rituals, can restore natural balance and improve sleep quality.**

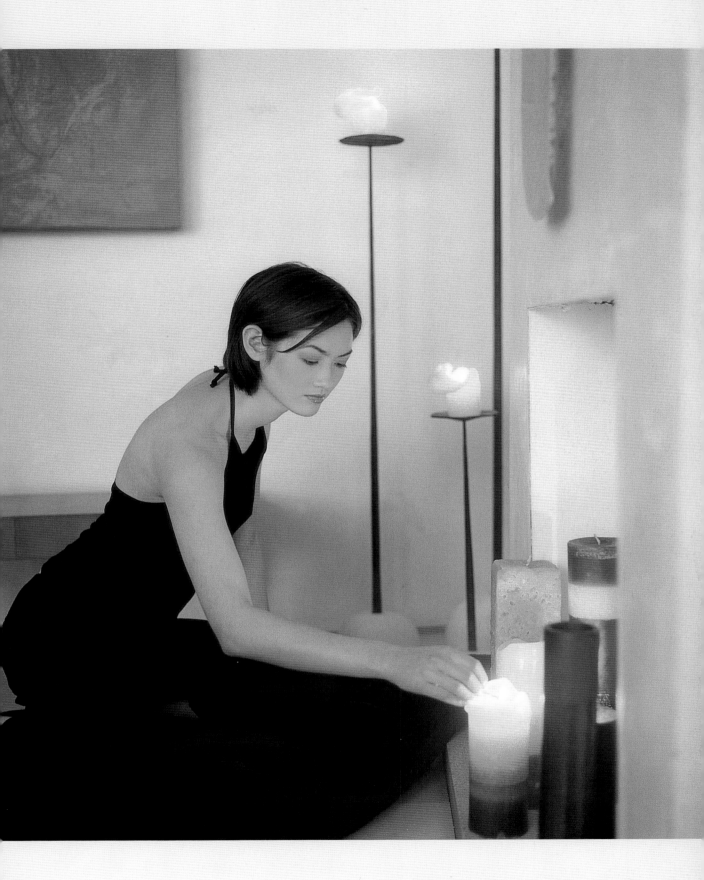

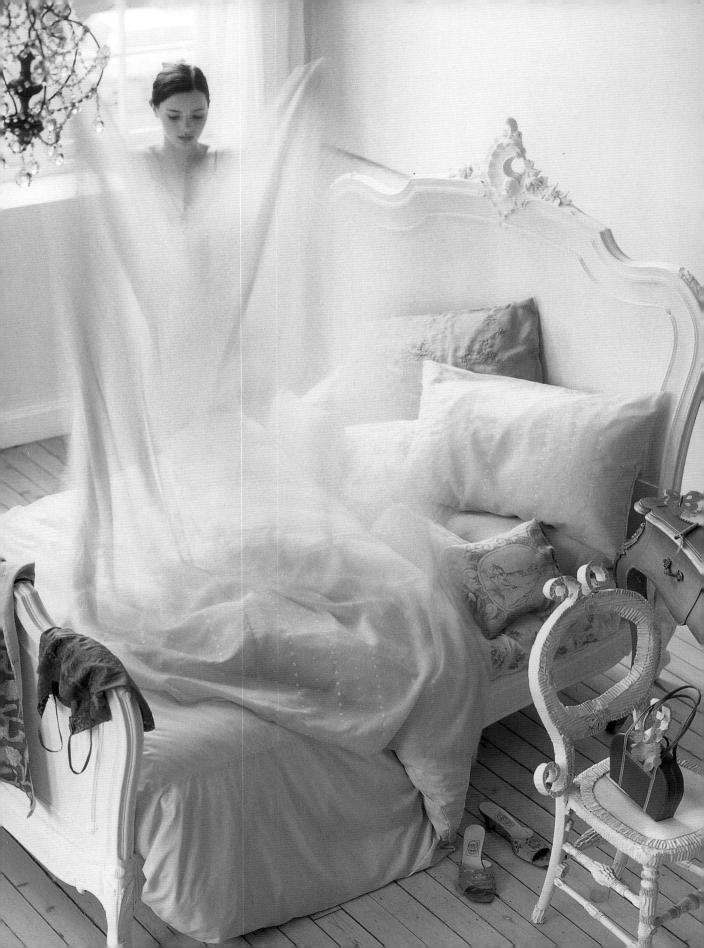

2 Assessing Your Sleep Problems

WE ALL KNOW HOW IT FEELS to be sleepy, and how coping with the following day's stresses and strains can feel like you are wading through molasses, but most of us underestimate the far-reaching effects of sleep deprivation. From waking, you may find the transition into daytime mode more difficult to make. You feel sluggish and disorientated, and simple tasks, such as making breakfast, may take longer to perform.

You may find yourself much more irritable and snappy with anyone who has the misfortune to cross your path. Added to this, you may also feel a sensation of light-headedness and your coordination is impaired – this is when you stub your toe or spill your coffee!

Other changes in mood, such as sadness and lack of emotional resilience, become apparent. You may become emotionally detached and, slowly, all your communication, social and memory skills start to deteriorate. Overtired people lose their ability to make clear decisions and, as a result, often exhibit poor judgement by making snap decisions. Some of the biggest manmade disasters of the last century were believed to be a result of human fatigue – the 1986 Chernobyl nuclear reactor accident; the capsizing of the passenger car ferry *Herald of Free Enterprise* in the Belgian port of Zeebrugge; and the 1997 Korean Air flight 801,

which crashed killing 228 people. Paranoia, aggression and apathy may also make an appearance, which can obviously have serious effects on personal relationships.

Excessive sleep deprivation has quite radical effects on the body. Experiments have shown that animals will eventually die if they are kept constantly awake, so it can be assumed that it would have a similar effect on humans. From sleep deprivation experiments conducted on human beings, we know that the body will begin to exhibit the following range of symptoms, to some degree, after only a few days without sleep:

- Dry, itchy eyes
- Increased appetite
- Bad skin
- Impaired vision
- Chapped lips
- Increased pain sensitivity
- Drop in body temperature
- Disturbed breathing patterns.

You can liken the effects of being tired to being drunk. Going without sleep for only 21 hours is the

LEFT Although a poor night's sleep makes everyone feel similarly dreadful, the actual reasons for sleep problems can be numerous and varied.

equivalent to having 0.8 per cent alcohol in your system, which is over the legal limit to drive in many countries. As well as the physical similarities to being drunk, such as swaying and bumping into things, when you are tired you may also lose your social inhibitions, act overconfident or behave badly without any embarrassment, and be unable to communicate properly, including losing interest in sentences halfway through. Strangely, you may also experience an increase in libido, although no one knows quite why.

BELOW **Our 24-hour culture offers us endless temptations to cut back on our sleeping hours, and few good reasons to have an early night.**

TYPES AND CAUSES OF INSOMNIA

Although most people associate the term insomnia with endless nights lying awake staring into the gloom, waiting to drop off, it is actually a catch-all term used to describe a wide variety of symptoms with varying degrees of severity and covering problems such as staying asleep or waking up too early in the morning. Each of these disorders requires a different type of treatment, and determining whether or not you are suffering from primary or secondary insomnia is the first step to receiving the appropriate one.

Primary insomnia is classified as disturbance to sleep patterns lasting at least a month and has no obvious physical or medical cause. Secondary insomnia is a side effect of a separate complaint,

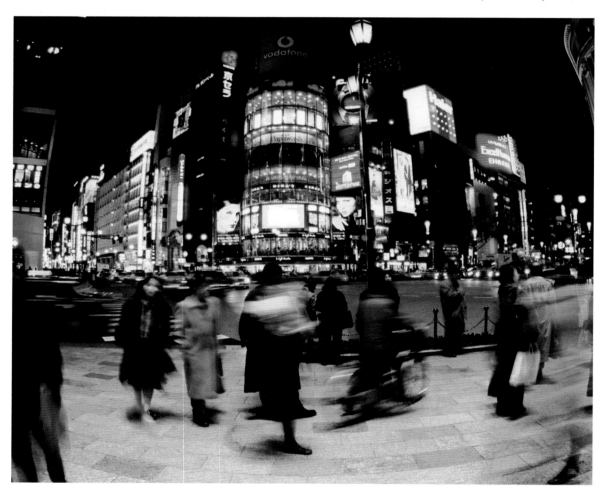

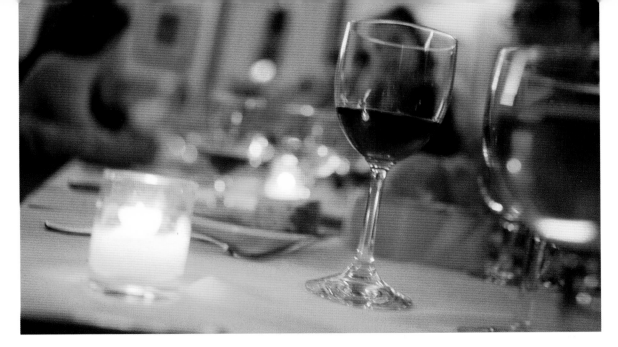

ABOVE **Alcohol is one of several stimulants that gives us an initial energy boost, but that ultimately affects our ability to get a good-quality night's sleep.**

such as asthma (which can worsen at night, causing sleeplessness) or depression.

Causes for the insomnia are classified as intrinsic (a condition within the body, such as sleep apnoea, narcolepsy or Restless Leg Syndrome) or extrinsic (such as alcohol-disturbed sleep, a noisy sleeping environment or an emotional complaint, such as stress or grief). And the length is also key in deciding how serious your problem is: transient insomnia is a disturbance in sleeping patterns that lasts for a few nights, brought on by factors such as jet lag, excitement, stress, illness or a change in sleep schedule. Intermittent insomnia persists for about two to three weeks, and can be caused by a job change, serious illness or financial problems. Chronic insomnia lasts longer than a few weeks and seems to show no signs of abating naturally; perhaps the cause is unclear.

When trying to treat insomnia, you need first to understand which of these categories your symptoms fall into; this will then help you to find the key to restoring restful sleep. A good way to work out the cause of your poor sleep is to keep a sleep diary, to help pinpoint any recurring themes. If you can track a pattern, such as deadlines and late dinners directly affecting your ability to drop off, you can start by eliminating them, or managing them differently; in some cases, simply moving the TV out of the bedroom can have startlingly effective results (see also pages 58–70).

However, self-help measures may not bring you any real relief. It may be that you are suffering from a condition called psychophysiological insomnia, which describes 'learnt' insomnia. A period of sleeplessness may have been triggered by grief or stress, and can persist long after the negative event has been dealt with. Or the sleeper can have become anxious about sleeping well, making it a source of stress and stimulus in itself. Idiopathic insomnia describes a life-long sleeplessness that is usually attributed to an abnormality in the neurological or neurochemical control of the sleep-wake cycle, and usually makes itself known from childhood. There is also sleep state misperception, where a patient imagines they have slept much less than they actually have, but this can still leave them feeling dreadful and distressed.

Even if you need to approach a healthcare practitioner to address the problem, the diary will be invaluable in finding a treatment to fulfil your specific needs. It will also help ease the feelings of helplessness and frustration that so often accompany insomnia.

INTRINSIC INSOMNIA: WHEN THE BODY WORKS AGAINST US

In this section we will look at the most common complaints of 'intrinsic' insomnia, from body clock problems and snoring to more serious conditions.

Clocked Off

When our body clock works well, we feel sleepy when it is dark and ready to take on the day when there is daylight. However, this isn't always the case, and there are certain types of insomnia that are related directly to our circadian rhythm.

Those who find themselves fighting to keep their eyes awake as soon as dinner is over may be suffering from advanced sleep phase syndrome (ASPS). This is not merely a 'larks' tendency to go to bed early so they can enjoy their preferred 6 am start; it often has sufferers fighting a ridiculously early bedtime, as they know that they will find themselves wide awake, having had their full quota of eight hours, at 2 am. Their sleep is often refreshing, but simply out of step with the rest of their lives (and those around them). Resetting the circadian rhythm may be necessary using light therapy and 'chronotherapy', which moves the bedtime back gradually until they return to their normal pattern. This can also be helpful when tackling jet lag (by gradually adapting your bedtime to the new destination before you begin your journey).

The opposite syndrome is delayed sleep phase syndrome (DSPS). This is defined as the inability to fall asleep within two hours of our desired sleep time. It can often be exacerbated by the anxiety caused by knowing that one has to rise early for work. Both can be accompanied by depression as a result of the frustration and isolation they can cause. Light therapy and chronotherapy are again used to try to reset the body clock, and melatonin (see page 57 for details of how to use it) is also a good tool for encouraging the onset of sleep.

Another common form of insomnia, is para-somnias, which are disorders that disrupt sleep. The sufferer may fall asleep easily, only to wake fitfully as the night goes on. Partial awakening at night is part of the general sleep experience, but these disorders leave the sleeper feeling disturbed and worn out. They can include teeth grinding (bruxism), night terrors (wakening from a nightmare state screaming), bedwetting, sleep talking and somnambulism (movement while asleep, which also includes sleepwalking). Some are fairly harmless, and most of us experience them at some point, but all these conditions, if causing serious disruption, can be eased by a medical professional. For some it is as simple as a mouth guard from the dentist to prevent jaw pain from teeth grinding, or positive visualization techniques performed while awake to 're-plot' bad dreams; so suffering in silence is not necessary.

Snoring

The most common intrinsic (extrinsic to your partner) complaint, but by no means the less disruptive, is snoring. Anyone who lives with a snorer can tell you how draining and frustrating this can be. Some people snore so loudly that they even wake themselves up. Snoring affects around 3.5 million people in Britain, according to the British Snoring and Sleep Apnoea Association, and it is mostly men who snore. Men have thinner air pipes than women, but both lose muscle tone as they age, which makes us more susceptible to snoring as we get older. The good news is that 99 per cent of snoring cases can be treated.

Snoring occurs when the soft palate tissue at the back of the throat relaxes too much and obstructs the entrance to the throat. As air tries to pass through, the soft palate vibrates and produces the snoring sound. Alcohol can aggravate the symptoms as it is a muscle relaxant (sleeping pills can have the same effect). Another factor that can

RIGHT **A dysfunction in the natural body clock can mean sufferers get out of step with the rest of the world, forcing them to retire to bed very early or very late.**

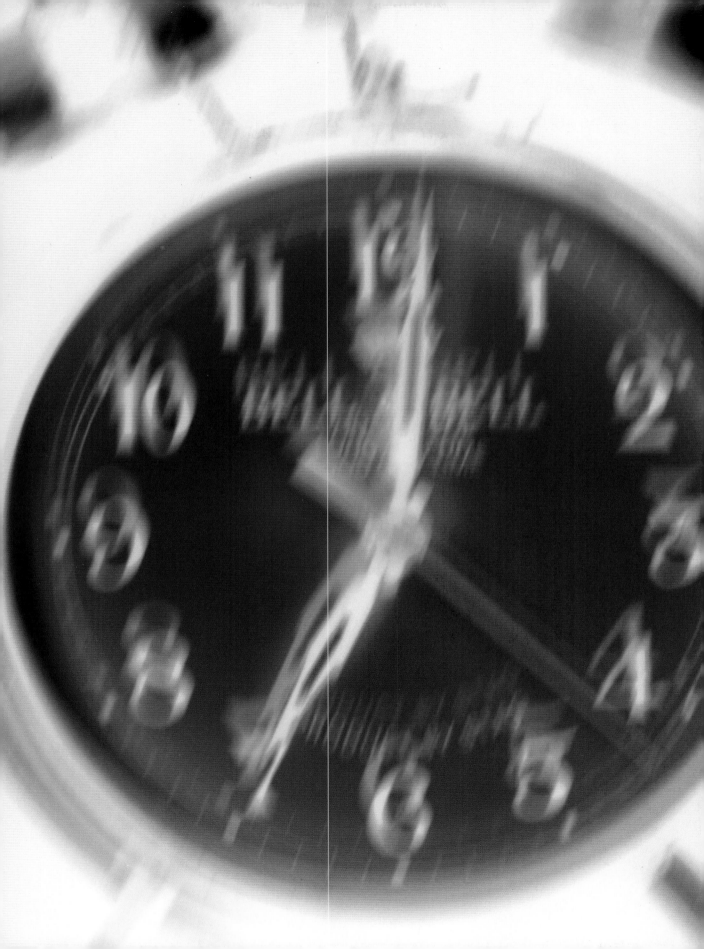

make snoring worse is excess body weight. People with a collar size of more than 42 cm (16½ inches) are more likely to snore because of the extra weight on their throat muscles. Snoring can also be caused by nasal congestion; avoiding dehydrating drinks like coffee, tea and alcohol, using a humidifier or putting eucalyptus oil on your pillow can help clear the passageways.

For most snorers, sleeping on the back exacerbates the problem, as the tongue falls backwards into the throat, which can narrow the airway and partly block airflow. Try sleeping on your side. If this doesn't work, pillows designed to help prevent snoring, losing weight to reduce pressure on airways, and even a mandibular device, which you wear like a mouth guard at night to bring the lower jaw forward and open up the airway at the back, can all help.

Sleep Apnoea

Apnoea is caused by the same muscles that cause snoring, but it is more dangerous because it alters normal breathing patterns. While asleep, sufferers may stop breathing for between 10 and 25 seconds at a time. This depletes the bloodstream and deprives the brain of vital oxygen supplies, which makes it suddenly send out an emergency signal, telling the person to wake up and take in a big gulp of air. In a single night sufferers may experience up to 350 apnoeic events and usually find themselves waking up sweaty, with a dry mouth and a head-ache. Sleep apnoea can be a potentially life-threatening condition, associated with strokes, heart attacks and high blood pressure, and therefore requires medical attention.

A sleep test called polysomnography is usually carried out to diagnose sleep apnoea. Mild cases can be effectively treated through lifestyle changes

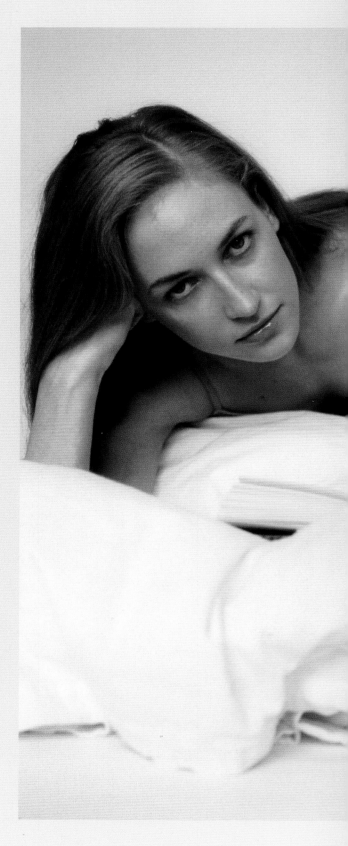

RIGHT **Insomnia can be infectious; sharing a bed with someone who suffers from snoring or sleep apnoea can ruin the sleep quality of both partners.**

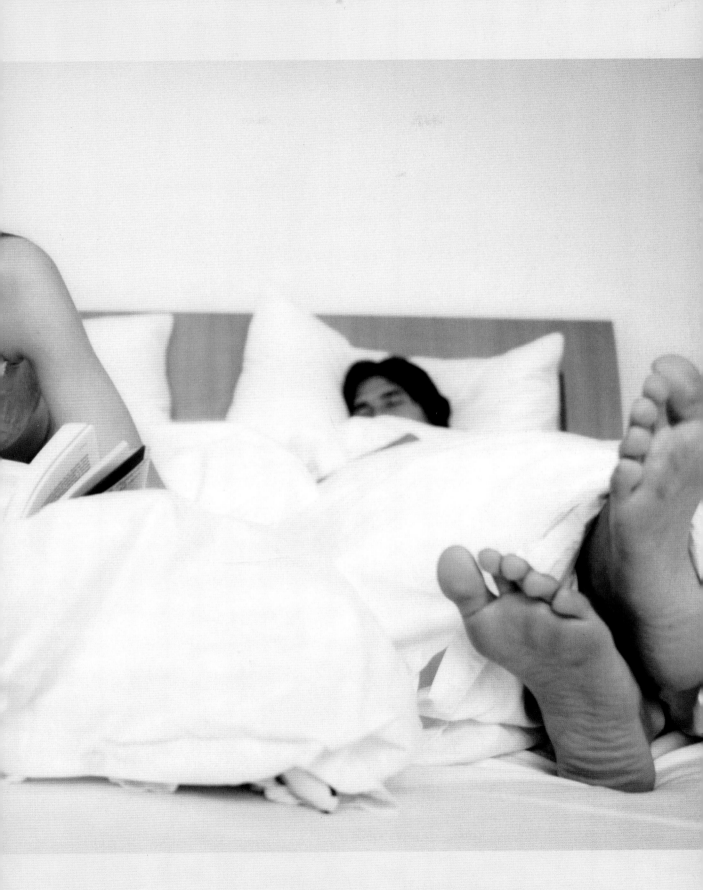

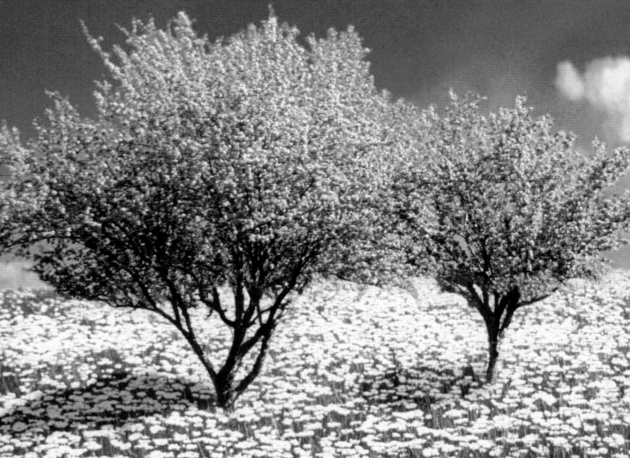

– losing weight, cutting down on alcohol or sleeping on your side, for example. More severe cases, which have been cited in some heart and respiratory failure fatalities, demand medical intervention, such as observation in a sleep clinic, or the prescription of a continuous positive airway pressure (CPAP) device, which supports your breathing at night.

Restless Leg Syndrome (RLS)

This condition is mainly associated with old age but it can strike at any time. RLS causes a tingling, itching or burning sensation and unexplained aches and pains in the lower limbs. The problem ranges from being simply uncomfortable to painful. Sleep is disturbed because people often have a strong urge to move the legs to relieve the discomfort by stretching, rubbing the legs or getting up and pacing around. It may be inherited, but hormonal changes during pregnancy may also worsen these symptoms. Caffeine and alcohol aggravate the sensations, so should be avoided. Massaging the legs, using a hot or cold pack, leg stretches, magnesium and iron supplements, and a warm bath can all help ease the symptoms.

A similar disorder that impairs sleep, periodic limb movement in sleep (PLMS) is characterized by involuntary leg twitching or jerking movements during sleep that typically occur every 10 to 60 seconds, sometimes throughout the night.

Narcolepsy

Most people think that a narcoleptic suffers from a condition that makes them fall asleep at random intervals, but narcolepsy can describe cataplectic attacks where people have physical symptoms of sudden sleep, such as collapsing, but are actually wide awake. An attack is often brought on by

LEFT **Many people suffer from a lack of daylight in the winter months, which increases their tendency to sleep for longer hours and to feel depressed.**

intense emotions, such as anger or sexual arousal. One person in a thousand suffers from narcolepsy and there are various causes – it can be a result of a head injury, a virus or an autoimmune disease. It can be accompanied by headaches, lethargy and poor concentration and, although hard to diagnose, it requires medical attention to find techniques that will help the sufferer and their loved ones to cope better.

A similar condition is known as hypersomnia, which is long-term excessive daytime tiredness with no clear cause. It is like narcolepsy but sufferers go into long phases of deep sleep, which can last up to two hours at a time. Occasional patches of hypersomnia can happen several times a day with periods without problems in between. Excessive tiredness can also happen after periods of intense stress on the body or emotions; this is known as post-traumatic tiredness.

Seasonal Affective Disorder (SAD)

As the winter nights begin to draw in, many people find themselves sleeping longer, eating more and generally feeling low and lacking in motivation. Many of us may recognize these symptoms, as it is a common complaint, although the extent of the problem can vary between every sufferer. Treatment is usually in the form of light therapy, exposing the patient to a light source of about 2,500 lux (lux is the measurement of light – average room lighting is about 250–500 lux). The light mimics the effect of the sun, which is though to control the production of melatonin – one theory is that darkness means more production of melatonin, which makes us lethargic and depressed. The best way to control this ourselves is to make the most of any available light by taking a daily walk outside. Also make sure that your curtains and blinds are wide open when the sun is out. Use brighter, daylight bulbs in your home to kickstart your daily cycle and get a 'sunlight' alarm clock to help your body prepare for the day. Also consider changing your annual holiday; two weeks in the sun in winter could perk you up dramatically.

Anxiety

Ranging from a nervous feeling when awaiting news to a full-blown, physical panic attack, anxiety can be terribly debilitating. It may have a reasonable cause, such as financial or personal uncertainties, but the symptoms may persist long after the initial trigger has been resolved – and this is known as 'free-floating anxiety'. It may even be that an unpleasant sleep association has developed, making the process of trying to get some much-needed – and healing – rest traumatic, and resulting in sleepless nights, which makes things seem even more unbearable and the chances of recovering without help less likely.

THE HAMILTON ANXIETY SCALE

If you have anxiety disorder, your doctor may use a special list of questions or statements to measure your symptoms. A popular one is the Hamilton Anxiety Scale. This scale lists 14 types of symptoms. You and your doctor rate each symptom on a scale from zero (meaning you don't have that symptom) to four (meaning you have it very badly). The total score can range from zero to 56. A total score of 18 or more means you should seek treatment for an anxiety disorder.

1 Anxiety, including worry, insecurity, irritability, fear, dread and panic.

2 Tension, including nervousness, muscle tension and trembling.

3 Fears, such as fear of enclosed spaces or fear of open spaces, and avoidance of these situations.

4 Lack of sleep or poor sleep.

5 Poor concentration or difficulty making decisions.

6 Depression, including sadness, gloom and hopelessness.

7 Muscle pain or weakness.

8 Trouble hearing, poor vision or unusual sensations on your skin (such as prickling).

9 Symptoms affecting your heart, such as palpitations (you feel your heart beating faster than normal) or feeling faint.

10 Trouble breathing.

11 Constipation, diarrhoea, nausea or other problems with your digestive system.

12 Needing to urinate too often; abnormal periods.

13 Nervous symptoms, such as sweating, dizziness or a dry mouth.

14 Feeling anxious, nervous or agitated while talking to your doctor.

As with depression, which is closely related and often accompanies anxiety, talking to a counsellor, practitioner or even a friend will help relieve the symptoms and speed the recovery process.

Depression

Sleep disorders and depression are frequent bedfellows. It can take many forms, such as being unable to fall asleep, waking frequently in the night or incredibly early or sleeping a disproportionate amount of time. Other symptoms may include a sense of hopelessness, weight loss, withdrawal from social interaction, fatigue, feelings of guilt, low libido, negative thought patterns, indecision and lack of focus. Some sufferers also have suicidal thoughts. It can vary in its intensity and duration and affects twice as many men as women.

Depression is treatable, so if the insomnia is a direct result of the illness, it can also disappear as soon as the treatment becomes effective. One of the main problems with depression is persuading sufferers that their feelings of shame regarding their situation are part of the condition and that, with treatment, they can begin to enjoy life again.

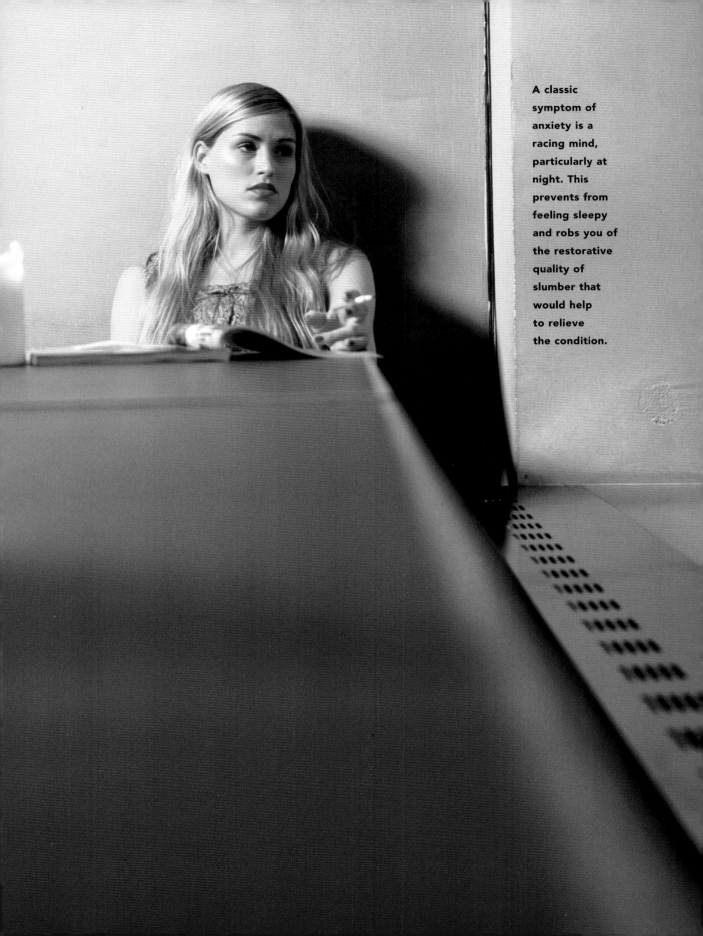

A classic symptom of anxiety is a racing mind, particularly at night. This prevents from feeling sleepy and robs you of the restorative quality of slumber that would help to relieve the condition.

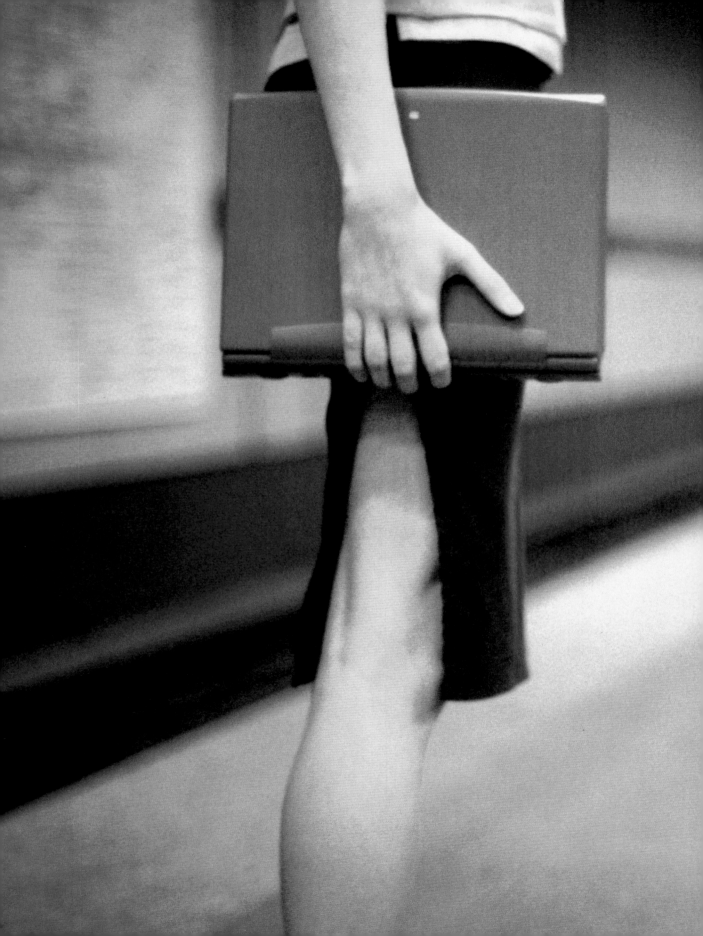

EXTRINSIC INSOMNIA: A LIFESTYLE OVERHAUL

Extrinsic insomnia is likely to affect us all at some point. According to research by the Better Sleep Council, 65 per cent of American adults claim they are losing sleep through stress. Stress itself can take many forms, but it mostly results in some form of constant low-grade sleep deprivation. Some life events cause a 'natural' insomnia, such as a new baby, menopause, the death of a loved one or illness. That is not to say that it is any more easy to cope with, but it is an expected part of these life-changing events and should rebalance in time, although you can help the situation along. Other forms of insomnia, or the creation of a sleep deficit from sleeping for too short a time, need treating at the root of the problem. Life in the fast lane and pressure at work demand a re-evaluation of your way of living.

The way we sleep changes constantly, with the amount we need gradually decreasing throughout our lives. For women, sleep patterns change throughout the month; the best sleep occurring immediately after menstruating and the worst in the run up to it. Pregnant women also experience a change in sleep patterns. They have more REM sleep and may find it hard to get comfortable or need to urinate in the night. Even women taking the oral contraceptive pill will have more shallow sleep than a woman using another form of contraceptive.

Work-Life Balance

In the current work culture, where we are expected to show our commitment through long hours and demanding schedules, it is easy to feel that we have no choice but to fall into line at the expense of our personal lives. But next time you decide to work into the small hours, consider the fact that you are less able to think laterally and creatively when you are tired. So those extra hours trying to come up with an idea, when your body is sagging and your mind wandering, would really be better spent

LEFT **Commuting, long hours and demanding schedules can make us feel that we have no choice but to cut back on unproductive sleeping hours.**

sleeping. Some scientists even believe that sleeping helps to filter out all the useless information of the day and helps us to process the more important stuff; a theory that might be supported by anyone waking up with the solution to a nagging problem they couldn't resolve the day before. The lack of interest and motivation that results from sleep deprivation has led to some US companies encouraging executives to take naps during the day to refresh themselves, and make them more focused. This policy is certain to see results, as a nap can instantly sharpen your powers of concentration.

Shift Work

Working shift hours is the result of our demand for a 24-hour society. Those caring for an elderly or sick friend or relative may experience similar sleep patterns to those doing shift work. The very existence of the 'darkness' hormone melatonin, which is produced at night to tell us to go to bed, is a clear sign that we are not nocturnal creatures. People who work shifts for a number of years are more likely to suffer from depression, heart disease and certain cancers, such as breast cancer in women. According to family physician and author Dr Paul Caldwell, switching from one shift to another is the most disruptive form of shift work; sticking to the same shift is much easier to cope with. The usual problems that flow from sleep deprivation, such as impaired personal relationships, becoming increasingly accident-prone and suffering from a suppressed immune system, all apply here; even though you are virtuously working away, the body makes no distinction. There are, however, some ways to make shift work more bearable.

Shift workers, or those catching a flight that will take them into a radically different time zone, can seriously benefit from a pre-emptive nap, which will help them cope with the changes and make them more alert and effective. Even if you still feel just as tired, research has shown that performance and adaptability is improved by a nap. For additional tips, see the box above and pages 38–9 on jet lag.

Tips for Surviving Shift Work

- When you are working, make sure the light is bright, and when you are meant to be sleeping, make sure the room is dark.

- Don't wait until the night you start your shift to change your sleeping patterns. Try to go to bed a little later each night in order to anticipate the change it will make to your wake-sleep patterns.

- Try to get 'power naps', especially if your job involves making important decisions. Even a 15-minute nap can sharpen your decision-making process.

- Make nutrition central to your wellbeing. Shift workers often resort to convenience food and alcohol to help them to wind down. Your body will cope better if you have nourishing meals.

- Make sure your partner or friends understand the toll on your system and emotions. It will help keep your relationships on track.

Stress

Everyone has some stress in their life. At best, it can motivate us to achieve our goals and respond to constantly changing demands; in its worst form it can give us horrible symptoms such as anxiety, depression, guilt, isolation, back pain, insomnia and headaches. Learning to manage our reaction to stress is essential to achieving a good night's sleep. In terms of feeling good, American women identify getting a good night's sleep as their top priority for personal wellness. The US Better Sleep Council discovered that 27 per cent believe that sleep is more important to wellness than eating a balanced diet (24 per cent) and exercising for 30 minutes a day (19 per cent). However, while 45 per cent of women say they feel most energized after a good night's sleep, only 16 per cent say that they are likely to sleep more to improve their overall wellness. Most people still leave sleep at the bottom of their priority list.

The main problem with stress is that it demands quick solutions. We tend to use quick fixes, such as caffeine, chocolate and processed snacks and meals, to make us feel instantly better so that we can get on top of the demands made of us. Finding time to buy nourishing fresh food or to do calming exercises can often seem totally implausible, but finding time to do them is vital if we are to arrive at a place where we can enjoy challenges and adapt to them, rather than feel desperate.

THE DAY-TO-DAY EFFECTS OF STRESS

The effects of poorly managed stress on the mind and body are wide ranging. The general, most noticeable symptoms are listed below.

The Symptoms of Stress

- Muscular tension, especially in the jaw, neck and shoulders
- Insomnia
- Poor concentration
- Infections, such as colds
- Lack of appetite
- Loss of sex drive
- Panic attacks
- Depression
- Low self-confidence
- Inability to make decisions
- Mood swings
- Inability to change thought patterns
- Digestion problems, such as constipation, diarrhoea
- Anxiety
- Headaches, dizziness or light-headedness
- Hyperventilation
- Palpitations
- Heartburn
- Tingling sensations on the skin
- Exacerbation of skin complaints, such as psoriasis, eczema and acne.

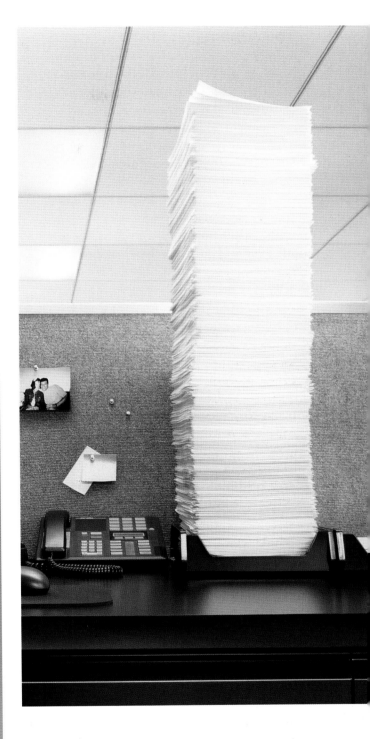

ABOVE **Learning to set boundaries when faced with a seemingly endless amount of work will greatly relieve the effects that stress has on sleep quality.**

The Adrenaline Rush

Every time we find ourselves faced with a new challenge, our body activates the 'fight or flight response'. The intensity of this reaction can depend on the type of situation we are in. The part of the autonomic nervous system that kicks into action is called the 'sympathetic' branch. It increases our rate of breathing, heartbeat, perspiration and production of the stress hormones cortisol and adrenaline and sends blood to muscles while shutting down our digestive system. We find ourselves with a sharpened mental awareness and a surge of physical energy and tension – this is what helps us to act quickly or meet that deadline. Once things have calmed down again, the 'parasympathetic' branch comes into play. This slows down all the mechanisms that speeded up and gets our digestion running again. Unfortunately, some people can start to rely on this 'rush' in order to get things done. This can have disastrous affects on long-term health and cause fatigue and exhaustion. Balancing the two systems is thus essential to our emotional and physical wellbeing. Repeatedly pushing ourselves past our limits will lead to burnout, a condition that will take far more than a few nights of extra rest to sort out.

Acknowledging our dependence upon these highs and the importance of taking control of our own state of mind is the first step to restoring a balance. Next, we need to make time to wind down through relaxation, visualization, meditation and breathing techniques, all of which can help us to drift off into a more refreshing sleep. We often assume that all our worries are valid rather than acknowledging that sometimes we may simply fall into negative patterns of thinking. Relaxing effectively is a learnt pattern of behaviour, in just the same way as negative thinking is, so why not choose the more pleasurable option?

Mastering relaxation techniques can have powerful physical and emotional impacts. If you find your concentration wandering to your 'to do' lists, start your recovery programme with an aromatherapy massage and let someone else

RIGHT **Preparing for the effects of jet lag and taking immediate steps upon arrival can greatly reduce stress on the body and help you adjust quickly to the new time zone.**

take over the technical side. Soon you will see the relaxing effects that such a practice can exert.

Jet Lag

Whether it's for pleasure or business, air travel is now common for many of us. While it may be a quick and convenient mode of travel, it also has its drawbacks. Jet lag, that awful 'travel hangover' that comes from skipping time zones, can wreak havoc with our body clocks and sleep patterns. Our bodies are designed to adjust to seasonal time changes, but not at the speed required when we travel across the world by aeroplane. The feelings of disorientation, nausea, headaches and insomnia are all a result of the disparity between the external indicators in our new destination conflicting with our body's expectation of where we are in our circadian rhythm cycle.

The reason we suffer more when travelling on an eastward flight is because the human biological clock lengthens its cycle, so that we can cope better with a longer day. When we travel east our day shortens and we lose time, making our sleep time less. Your body will still want to rest and you end up struggling not to sleep in the afternoon, when you should be at a meeting or, more importantly, out in the sun enjoying yourself. It has been estimated that the body adapts one hour a day when flying eastward, and one and a half on westward journeys. This is because our natural biological clock has a tendency to lengthen the day, so finds it easier to adjust to a longer day, which is what happens when we fly west (we 'gain' extra time). Travelling east, we 'lose' time, making our bedtime come too early (hence all that lying about feeling frustrated in our hotel room). So if you travel four hours east, it will take six days for you to feel fully recovered; travel six hours west and it only will take four.

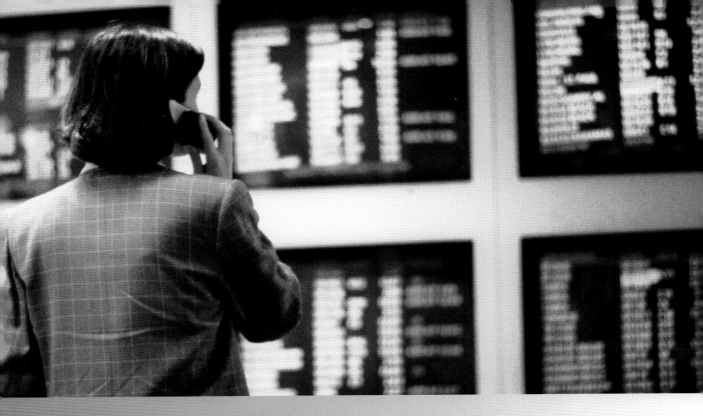

Tips for Enjoying a Restful Flight

What with jet lag, the noise, sleeping in the company of sometimes hundreds of strangers, children crying, cramped conditions, poor air quality, re-heated food and the general chaos and stress of the airport, there is very little to make you have a restful and refreshing journey.

Try some of the techniques listed below for making your recovery time shorter.

- **As soon as you get on the flight, make sure you change your watch to the new time and act accordingly – if it's 3 am at your destination, try to sleep.**
- **Don't wake up for the airline meals. Take your own snacks to eat at the right time, rather than just eating at a time that is convenient for the airline – more often than not, you won't be missing much!**
- **Eat well the day before the flight. Eat lots of fresh fruit, vegetables and lean protein so that your body is running at an optimum level to handle the stress.**
- **If you are travelling a long way, make changes in the week before you fly. Get up an hour later/earlier to adjust to the new time.**

- **Keep drinking water to help your body deal with the changes. Needless to say, dehydrating substances such as tea, coffee and alcohol won't help.**
- **Get out and about in daylight when you arrive. Lurking in the hotel room will only prolong the jet lag.**
- **Earplugs, eye masks and the reading light can help you make your own sun and moon. Use them to control your sense of the time of day.**
- **Do exercises, such as flexing and pointing your toes, stretching your arms above your head and walking around the plane, to help relieve muscle cramp and avoid Deep Vein Thrombosis (DVT).**
- **Natural sleep preparations can help if you need to sleep on the plane but also use carbohydrates to help you reach a soporific state.**
- **Vitamin B complex can help your body to cope with the strain of flying. Take it when you don't want to sleep, as it can be stimulating to the brain.**
- **When you arrive, use a power nap (no more than 90 minutes) to refresh your brain, and then get on with the day, no matter how much your body pleads for bed.**

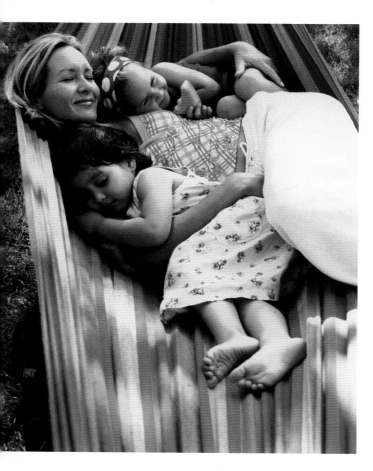

LEFT **All parents can testify to the chaos a new family member can inflict on your sleep patterns. Knowing what to expect, however, can help you to see the light at the end of the tunnel.**

he/she is drowsy, not asleep, with their face and head clear of blankets and other soft items.

3–11 MONTHS

When infants are put to bed drowsy but not completely asleep, they are more likely to become 'self-soothers', which enables them to fall asleep independently at bedtime and send themselves back to sleep if they wake during the night. After six months, infants may experience separation anxiety, but by this time many will sleep through the night, for about 9–12 hours with naps during the day.

1–3 YEARS

The standard sleep time at this age is 12–14 hours, with one long nap during the day of between one and three hours. Nightmares, the ability to get out of bed and separation anxiety can all make sleep difficult. A security blanket or stuffed toy should help, as will firm enforcement of the sleep ritual.

3–5 YEARS

Children will sleep between 11 and 13 hours a night by this age, although falling asleep and waking is common. Sleepwalking and sleep terrors may peak at this time. Maintaining a sleep schedule that ends in a cool, dark room should help.

5–12 YEARS

Daytime naps should end about this time. Children aged five to 12 need 10–11 hours of sleep, but there are now increasing demands on their waking time from school and social schedules. Watching TV close to bedtime has been associated with bedtime resistance, difficulty falling asleep and sleeping fewer hours. Make sure they don't have a TV in their bedroom, so that you can monitor how much they watch.

New Kid on the Block

A baby in the house is a joyous thing, but it can also have a profound impact on the sleep quality of everyone else. Understanding the sleep process and patterns of your growing child can help in this situation, but ultimately the best thing to remember is that each phase is just that, a phase. As difficult as it is to do, and sometimes it will not be practical or possible, try to sleep when your baby sleeps in the first few months. This will help refresh you and prevent exhaustion.

1–2 MONTHS

Newborns can sleep between 10½ and 18 hours a day and, as any new parent will tell you, at irregular hours. Exposing them to light and noise during the day can encourage them to sleep more at night. The National Sleep Foundation of America suggests putting the baby in the cot (crib) when

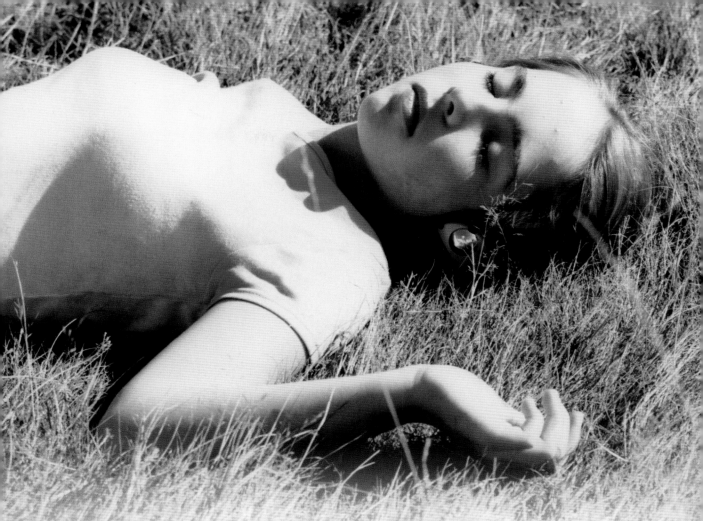

SERIOUS SLEEP PROBLEMS

Sometimes lifestyle stresses and worries are only a part of the issue when someone can't sleep. A significant number of sleep difficulties are caused by specific sleep disorders; according to the British Association of Counselling and Psychotherapy it is estimated that 25 per cent of the UK population suffer from some form of sleep disorder and it is believed that many more of these conditions remain untreated and undiagnosed.

TO SLEEP, PERCHANCE TO DREAM

In our time-pressured culture, sleep is often seen as a nuisance that gets in the way of more enjoyable or essential pasttimes. This may be work, but it is also often drinking, dancing and generally having fun. A good, rewarding sleep, however, can bring a great deal of pleasure in its own right.

ABOVE **Daytime fatigue due to sleepless nights need not be endured. Seeking out help will identify if you have a specific sleep disorder that can be treated.**

Sleep can impact positively on your personal relationships, making you relaxed and happy and helping you deal with stress by making you more emotionally prepared to cope with the strains of everyday living. This will help you to enjoy more of the life around you by keeping you sharp, alert and engaged. Your levels of creativity and mental agility are also fine-tuned by sleep, as is your immune system, which is boosted by sleep, keeps infection at bay and improves your resistance to disease. Don't forget that lovely warm feeling you get from waking from a restful night's slumber to a bright summer's morning, full of energy and ready to make the most of what the day has to offer.

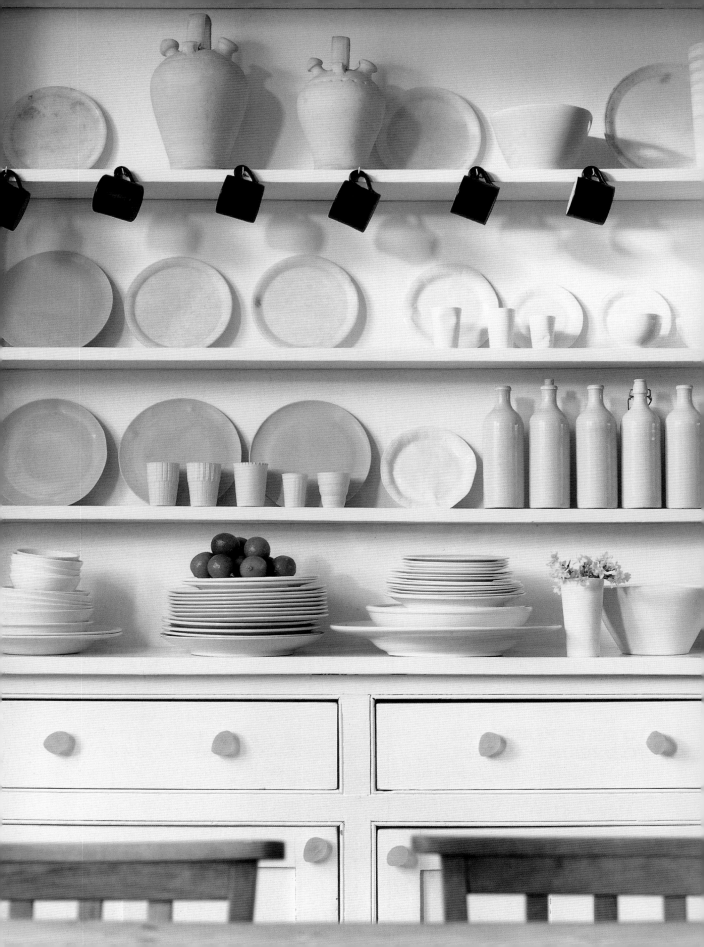

3 Food, Drink & Sleep

FOOD AND DRINK, LIKE SLEEP, are an essential part of living a healthy and fulfilling life, but we often forget that our body works as a whole. Most of us, for example, fail to acknowledge the effect that alcohol, caffeine and rich food might have on our patterns of sleep, and feel frustrated when we sleep the requisite amount of time yet don't feel refreshed.

In reality, most people are unwilling to live an entirely abstemious life. Try wrestling a cup of cappuccino from the hands of a caffeine addict just before they leave for work and you will begin to appreciate how many of us rely on such props to help us make it through the day. With that in mind, it's worth admitting your weaknesses and planning out your daily diet sensibly to avoid the food and drinks that keep you awake and to begin to appreciate more soporific foods later in the day.

SLEEP AND WEIGHT

For those trying to lose weight, good sleep could be essential. A recent study by Columbia University in New York indicates that there is a link between sleep and the US's obesity epidemic. The research suggests that the more you sleep, the less likely you are to become obese. People who get less than the recommended amount of sleep each night are up to 73 per cent more likely to be obese although,

LEFT What we put into our body during the day can greatly affect our ability to fall asleep at night, and also the quality of rest that follows.

obviously, obesity is also usually the result of several other lifestyle factors. It has also been proved that there is a connection between middle-aged spread in men and the quality of sleep they have. Men, during sleep, produce the growth hormone. This hormone maintains and renews muscle tone, but it decreases naturally with age, as does the amount of sleep men need. The problem is, if they don't fulfil their sleep needs, they won't be getting as much of the growth hormone as they could – thus speeding the arrival of a stomach paunch.

THE BAD STUFF

Caffeine, in beverages such as tea, coffee and fizzy drinks, will keep you awake well into the night if you let it, so you need to enjoy your last cup at least five hours before bedtime. The same goes for heavy, rich foods. Although scientists say that there are no direct chemical reasons why such foods should keep you awake, your digestive system still needs to break down the food. As this is one of the functions that the body shuts down during sleep, it can keep you up, or affect your sleep quality, until it has finished its work. So a rich meal with alcohol at 10 pm is not the best idea; neither are stimulating meals that contain spicy foods, onions or peppers, which can give you indigestion and delay the onset of sleep.

As a general rule, you should try to avoid the following foods late at night:

• Fatty foods may cause heartburn, which leads to difficulty in falling asleep and discomfort throughout the night.

• Foods containing tyramine (bacon, cheese, ham, aubergines (eggplant), pepperoni, raspberries, avocado, soy sauce, red wine) might keep you awake at night. Tyramine causes the release of norepinephrine, a brain stimulant.

Caffeine

This is the most widely used drug in the world, and probably the most socially acceptable, but its effect should not be underestimated. Reactions to caffeine differ depending on a person's sensitivity, but is safe to say that the older you are, the greater its effect. About 99 per cent of the caffeine contained in a drink will enter your bloodstream. On the

BELOW **Caffeine stays in the body long after we feel the initial boost in energy and improved concentration that it gives. Treat it with caution.**

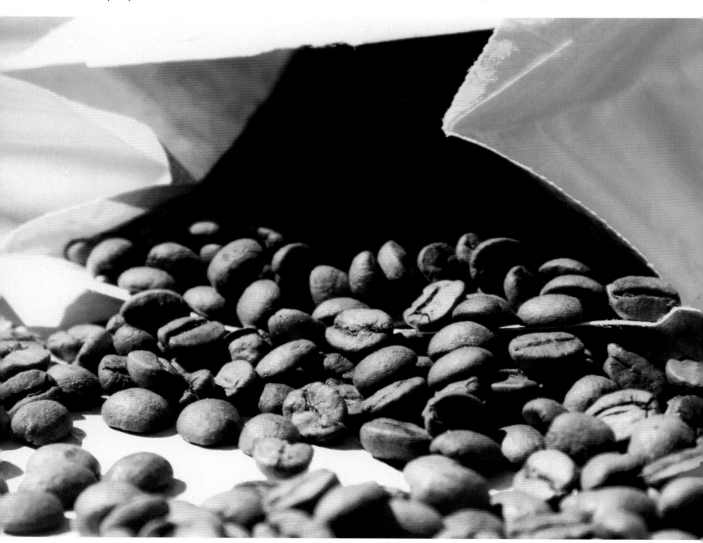

positive side, it can generate sensations of increased alertness and enhance performance in mental and physical tasks. On the negative side, it can create or exacerbate sensations of anxiety, depression, restlessness, headaches, flushes, tremors, heartburn and aggravate high blood pressure. It also has a profound effect on our ability to sleep, which is often the reason it is so popular in the first place.

Caffeine enters the blood stream quickly (in about five minutes) and its effects are felt for between 15 and 45 minutes. It then takes between three and seven hours for half of it to be filtered out of your blood stream. For most people, the remaining half is filtered out overnight, which is why addicts are often reaching for the coffee filters before they have even changed out of their pyjamas.

As well as your waking time, caffeine also effects your sleeping time. It suppresses feelings of sleepiness and pushes back the time you hit the pillow, in which case that last coffee or tea of your working day keeps you perky for much longer than you would often hope for. Remember that, as well as coffee and tea, caffeine is also found in cola drinks, chocolate, cocoa, energy drinks, and even some cold remedies and headache and painkillers. Make sure, if you do want to give up, that you don't just end up reaching for it in other forms.

LIFE AFTER CAFFEINE

If you believe that some of the symptoms caused by caffeine are affecting your quality of life, the good news is that caffeine leaves your system quickly. Detoxing from it might give you a nasty headache for a few days, with some irritability and nausea, but you should be able to cope. Increase your daily intake of water and fresh juices to help flush caffeine out, and deal with the temptation by making herbal tea instead; this means you won't have to miss out on the sensation of a comforting warm drink as you work or relax. If you would like to keep coffee as part of your daily life, give yourself a cut-off time of, say, noon to allow the caffeine adequate time to leave your system.

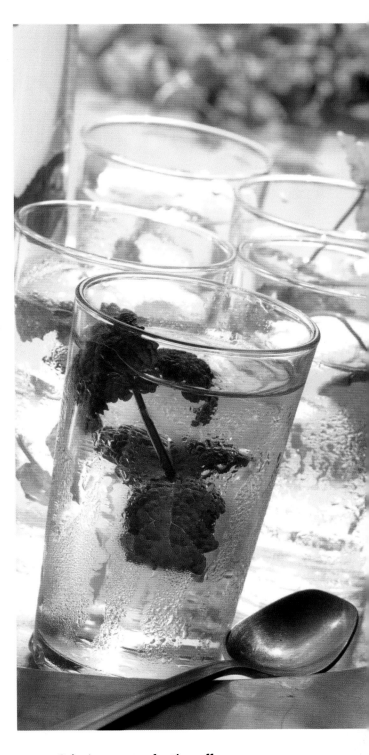

ABOVE **Substitute water for the coffee, tea and carbonated cola drinks in your diet – a sprig of mint or a little lemon or lime juice will make it less bland.**

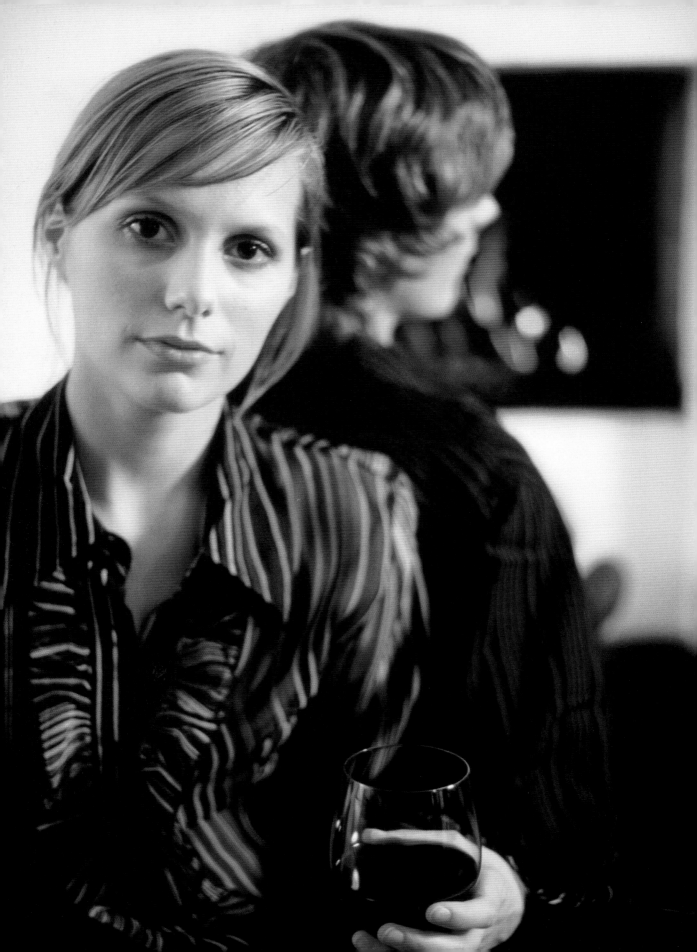

Nicotine

This is the largest preventable cause of death in our society, yet it still plays a huge part in many people's lives. It is a major cause of cancer in the lungs and heart, heart disease and high blood pressure – the risks are manifold. Smokers might cite suppressed appetite (they tend to be an average of 5–10 lb (2.2–4.5 kg) lighter than nonsmokers) and increased memory ability as bonuses, but the undisputed deterioration of their overall health is a high price to pay. Smokers might also note that the good sleep quality they lack thanks to the nicotine in their body could help them to maintain a good weight and memory recall without the health hazard. Unfortunately, the highly addictive nature of nicotine stops many people from acknowledging the risks. Like most drugs, the pleasant, calming sensation created after the initial intake can turn into a jittery, angst-ridden feeling if you don't keep the levels in your body up.

Smokers are statistically more likely to drink more caffeine, which only compounds the side effect of destroying sleep quality. Smoking also affects blood sugar levels, which makes you irritable and prone to sugar cravings. As a stimulant, nicotine acts on the central nervous system and delays sleep as well as increasing the frequency of night-time wakings, which results in a light and less refreshing sleep. Anyone who lives with a heavy smoker and suffers from poor sleep may also be experiencing the effects of passive smoking on their systems.

LIFE AFTER NICOTINE

Giving up is hard, but the health benefits will more than outweigh the effort you put in. When inhaled, nicotine quickly stimulates the heart, brain, gastro-intestinal tract and adrenal glands, giving the buzz or peak in alertness that comes with a drag on a cigarette. As it is a brain stimulant, it can stop the

LEFT **Although alcohol can often help you to fall asleep, it also makes you wake more frequently during the night.**

onset of sleep, but also increase the number of night-time wakings and shorten the duration of sleep; and remember, if it is affecting your sleep, it will affect that of your partner and children, too, as they passively inhale your smoke. Initially, those giving up smoking will experience disturbed sleep from the nicotine withdrawal, but patches and supplements can help ease this transition. Once you are past this point, you will be rewarded with a much deeper and nourishing sleep, as will anyone else in your home.

Alcohol

A great deal of self-deception is at work when people use the term 'nightcap' to describe alcohol. Although, as a sedative, it helps you to fall to sleep by making you feel drowsy, it then proceeds to ruin the rest of your night.

Drinking is a hugely popular aid to relaxation, especially for those working long and strenuous hours. Those who drink on an empty stomach will feel the sensation quicker, as drinking with or after food can delay its effects for up to an hour and a half. How tired you are when you start drinking is also important. After five nights of partial sleep deprivation, three drinks will have the same effect on your body as six would have on a regular night.

If you find the sedative effect more pronounced after drinking during the day, this is because it exaggerates the natural ebb and flow of your circadian rhythm. The energy lull you feel in the afternoon becomes more pronounced, whereas you are naturally more alert in the evening, so its drowsy effects are less dramatic.

We all know the general results of drinking, but its impact on sleep is often ignored. Even a small amount of alcohol can change the type of sleep quality we have. REM sleep and the length of sleep we have are reduced, with more wakings and shallow sleep, which results in an unrefreshing sleep. It also has a detrimental effect on sleep conditions, such as apnoea and snoring, making both more pronounced. Alcohol is also a diuretic, which means it encourages you to urinate, which is never welcome when you are trying to sleep.

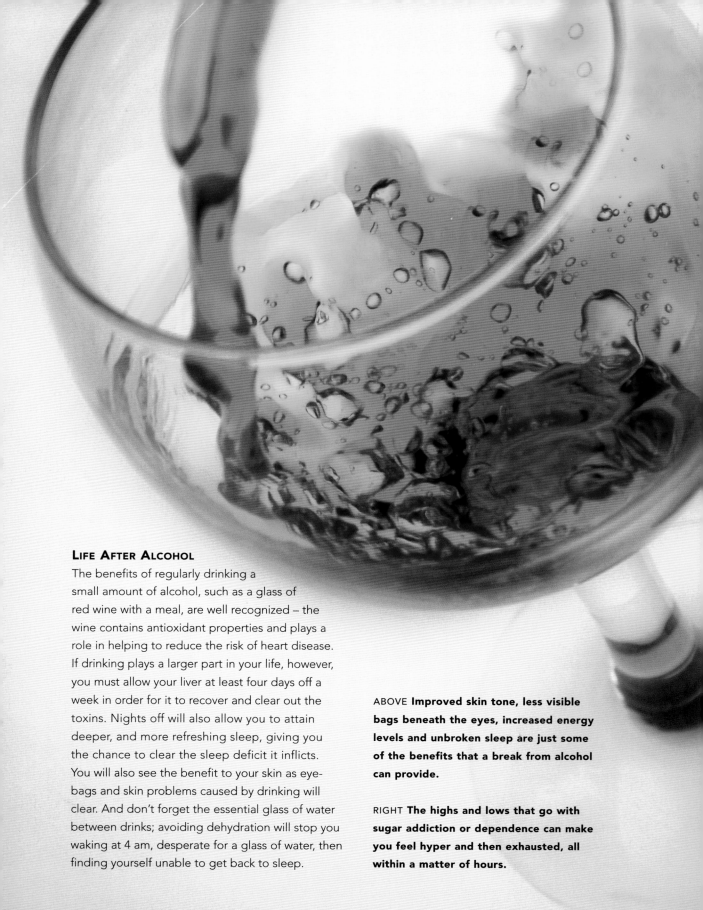

LIFE AFTER ALCOHOL

The benefits of regularly drinking a
small amount of alcohol, such as a glass of
red wine with a meal, are well recognized – the
wine contains antioxidant properties and plays a
role in helping to reduce the risk of heart disease.
If drinking plays a larger part in your life, however,
you must allow your liver at least four days off a
week in order for it to recover and clear out the
toxins. Nights off will also allow you to attain
deeper, and more refreshing sleep, giving you
the chance to clear the sleep deficit it inflicts.
You will also see the benefit to your skin as eye-
bags and skin problems caused by drinking will
clear. And don't forget the essential glass of water
between drinks; avoiding dehydration will stop you
waking at 4 am, desperate for a glass of water, then
finding yourself unable to get back to sleep.

ABOVE **Improved skin tone, less visible
bags beneath the eyes, increased energy
levels and unbroken sleep are just some
of the benefits that a break from alcohol
can provide.**

RIGHT **The highs and lows that go with
sugar addiction or dependence can make
you feel hyper and then exhausted, all
within a matter of hours.**

Sugar

In all its forms, sugar can play havoc with our sleep patterns. This is mainly because our blood sugar levels can 'crash' after a big dose of the stuff, leaving us even more tired, and hunting around for another snack to give us a quick energy fix, often washed down with our old friend caffeine. This cycle can leave us too fatigued to make a substantial dinner for ourselves, even if we feel ravenously hungry, and this is where convenience food comes in with even more hidden sugars and chemical sweeteners. And so the cycle continues.

LIFE AFTER SUGAR

Cutting down on sugar means committing to eating foods in their natural state. This means avoiding processed foods and weaning our sweet tooth on to more natural sugars, such as honey (in moderation). Balancing out the peaks and troughs of blood sugar can aid in weight loss, as we are not overeating and always hurtling from one unhealthy food fix to another, and balance our energy and concentration levels. This will mean you arrive at bedtime ready for a good night's sleep. The key to healthy snacking is to be prepared; a bag of roasted pumpkin seeds in your bag, a fruit bowl on your desk, will make them an easier option than finding a vending machine full of energy-sapping sugary and salty snacks. Aim to graze through the day rather than find yourself suddenly starving and willing to eat whatever you can find (it's always easier to find junk food). Little and often is best, and will stop you suddenly obsessing about what to have mid-morning.

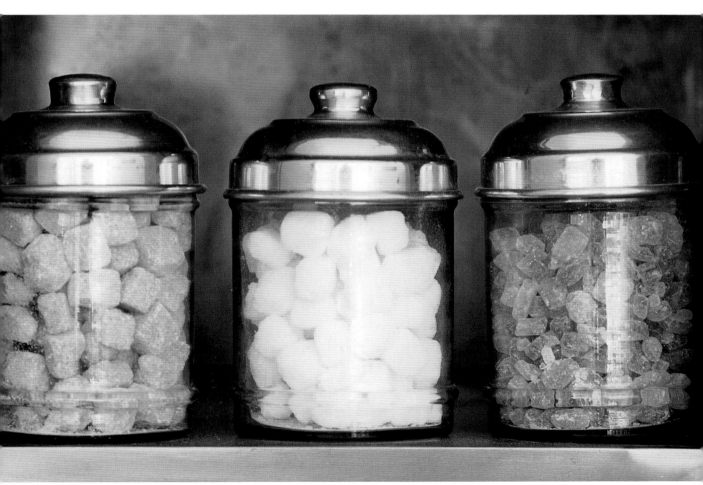

ENERGY-STABILIZING FOODS

The effect on mood and concentration from jolts in blood sugar can make coping with everyday problems more difficult. When the blood sugar level is raised, the pancreas produces insulin to bring it down again (and if this happens too often diabetes can develop). The short-term effect on our energy is to make us feel exhausted, irritable and stressed. We should choose foods that keep our energy levels at a fairly constant level, which helps us to concentrate and frees us from the urge to keep refuelling. It also improves our general mood, making us calmer and more balanced, so we are less likely to lie awake at night fretting over details or wound up from the caffeine in the emergency chocolate bar that we consumed before going to bed.

When looking for ingredients to create meals, keep in mind the following:

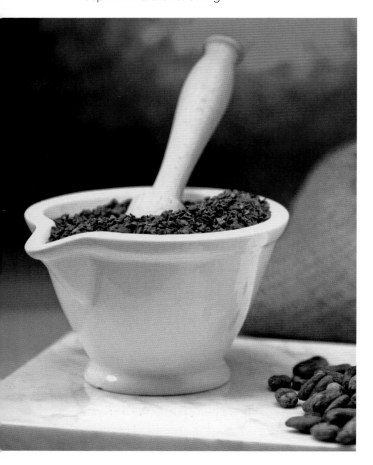

- Water aids digestion, so try to drink at least 2 litres (3½ pints) a day.

- Fresh fruit is the best slow-release energy source. Juicing fruit removes all the pulp and fibre, which stops you just getting a sugar hit from the fructose.

- Eating protein-rich foods, such as lean meats, cheese, eggs, natural yogurt and fish, for lunch will keep your levels balanced as you enter the natural dip in your circadian rhythm. Eating refined carbohydrates, like white bread, will cause your sugar level to soar then crash, and only exaggerate this natural dip.

- Pulses, beans, lentils, nuts and seeds are all great for slow-release energy – try them with wholegrain bread.

- Chromium-rich foods, such as shellfish, cheese, baked beans and wholegrain bread, help your body overcome extreme low blood sugar.

- A ravenous hunger the morning after a night of drinking is because the alcohol affects your blood sugar levels, making you reach for quick fixes the next day. Drinking on an empty stomach, makes it worse.

The Glycaemic Index

The body needs glucose for energy. It is obtained from starches and sugars in the food we eat and either used or stored as fat. Everything we eat is processed this way, but it is the speed at which this happens that makes the difference to our weight and general health – this is what gives food its GI rating. The faster food is broken down, the higher its index rating (a high rating is about 70 or above). Low-GI foods keep us fuller for longer, have more fibre, and are usually full of minerals and vitamins.

LEFT **To keep your energy levels stable, avoid stimulating food and drinks, such as coffee and chocolate. Although they may seem to improve your mental focus, they can cause mood swings.**

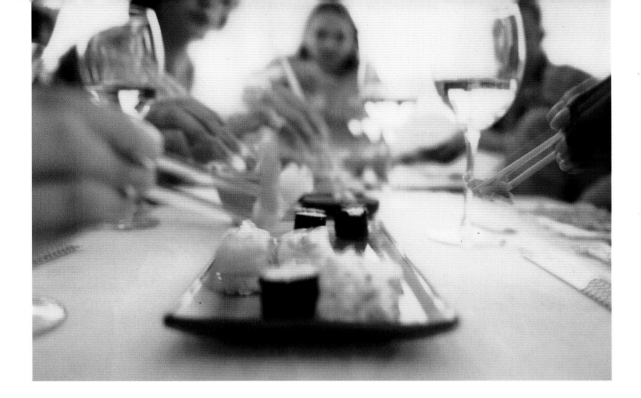

The lower the glycaemic index (GI) rating of food, the better it is for maintaining a balanced sugar level. Eating foods with a low GI rating, such as pulses, lentils and beans, is a great help when you are giving up stimulants such as caffeine and nicotine because they help prevent the swings in mood and hunger. The more processed food is, like white bread, white sugar and junk food, the higher it tends to be on the Index.

Choosing energy-balancing foods and drinks during the day can help you feel healthily tired and unwound by bedtime. A large breakfast of complex carbohydrates, such as porridge, fruit, nuts, seeds and lean protein will keep you balanced.

Tryptophan, the Insomniac's Friend

The good news is that for all the foods and drinks that overstimulate us and keep us awake at night, nature has provided sleep-inducing alternatives. Some calm us down while others actively deliver sedative effects. This is mainly down to a chemical called tryptophan.

Tryptophan is an amino acid and an essential chemical for life as it helps us to build protein. We consume about one to three grams of tryptophan a day, but we can boost our intake by seeking out

ABOVE **Learning to choose low-glycaemic index foods, such as sushi and sashimi, is simple. As a rule, avoid highly processed foods that are far removed from their original, natural state.**

foods that have a higher concentration. It has the effect of speeding up the onset of sleep, decreasing the number of spontaneous wakings during the night and increasing the overall length of sleep during the night. Elderly people, who suffer from increased sensitivity to noise, find it especially helpful, as do those on antidepressants because it can raise the level of serotonin, which is low in brains of depressed people. Eating a main meal around four hours before bedtime with a low-to-medium GI rating, including complex carbohydrates or some of the vegetables listed on page 52 will help start the relaxing process.

If needed, a tryptophan-rich snack before bedtime, such as the snacks listed on page 52, should greatly improve your chances of getting a good night's rest. Remember, however, that the same rules apply as before; make sure you give any snacks enough time to digest (an hour or so) before you go to bed.

Foods Rich in Tryptophan

- Bananas
- Turkey
- Milk and other dairy products
- Almonds
- Cabbage
- Kidney or lima beans
- Oats
- Poppy seed
- Pumpkin seed
- Spinach
- Wheat
- Evening primrose seed (contains the most tryptophan of any food source)
- Poultry
- Eggs
- Red meats
- Soybean
- Tofu
- Basil
- Dill

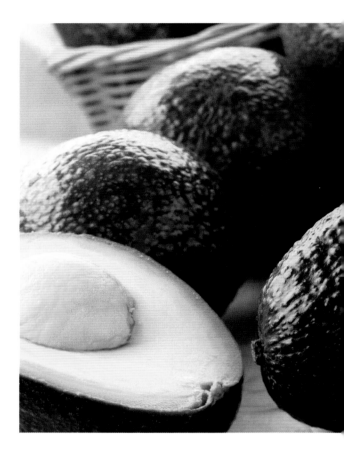

Sedative Snacks That Aid Relaxation Before Sleep

Combine 'sleepy food' with other foods, such as avocados, mandarins and lettuce that contain bromine to help ease that short-fused feeling, for a light, easy-to-make and easy-to-digest snack.

Lettuce has a longstanding reputation for promoting healthy sleep. This is due to an opium-related substance, combined with traces of the anticramping agent hyoscyarnin, that is present in lettuce. Lettuce should be an integral part of your evening diet if you are suffering from sleep disorders. Juiced, and mixed with a little lemon juice for flavour, it makes an effective sleep-inducing drink and is highly preferable to the synthetic chemical agents in sleeping pills. You can also try carbohydrates, including pasta, brown rice and oatmeal, which produce serotonin.

Try one of these delicious snacks an hour before bedtime to help you to relax and unwind:

ABOVE **Eating tryptophan-rich foods can help induce a restful and rewarding sleep in a completely natural way. Avoid stimulants and rich dishes before bedtime.**

RIGHT **Herbal drinks can settle the stomach, soothe the mind and relax the body. Try blending them for the perfect mix of taste and sensation for your individual needs.**

- Wholegrain toast with a little almond butter
- A small portion of a healthy, fat-containing food, such as olive oil on your salad or an avocado
- A small pot of natural yogurt with a little honey
- Fresh, dried or cooked fruit for dessert
- A small cup of warm milk, with nutmeg for flavour and digestion
- A small banana
- A handful of unsalted nuts or seeds.

Soothing Drinks

The traditional drink of a glass of warm milk before bedtime does indeed consist of calming properties – the tryptophan, calcium and magnesium all help the mind and body to relax. Try adding a sprinkling of cinnamon, which is excellent for digestion and can ease a sore throat or night-time cough.

Difficulties in breathing can sometimes be aggravated by dairy products, so consider other relaxing drink options. Herbal tea blends can be wonderful at sending you off to sleep; experiment with different blends to find your favourite.

PASSIONFLOWER

The passionflower vine is a sedative and digestive aid. The herb is considered to be a mildly effective treatment for anxiety and insomnia, and is often combined with other herbal preparations, such as valerian and hops. It isn't as potent as some of the other natural sedatives, but it is ideal for those who also get a nervous stomach, especially in the tea form, taken three times daily.

CAMOMILE

The familiar *camomilla* plant is used in varying degrees to help calm and relax. As well as being drunk, it can also be used to create a soothing, sleep-inducing bath before bedtime: simply put a teabag or two into the bath, or float some of the dried flowerheads in the water. Camomile is quite easy to grow if you fancy a constant supply – just dry it out and use. Add a little honey if you need a sweet kick, but not too much!

LEMON BALM

Also known as *Melissa officinalis*, this strong lemon-smelling member of the mint family can be made into tea. Also try using it to season soups and salads, or as a cooling iced tea on hot, restless summer nights.

VERBENA

Also known as lemon verbena, this is similar in flavour to lemon balm, but with a stronger taste, and has similar effects.

LIME FLOWER

Also known as linden, lime flower has soporific effects. Infuse a handful of dried flowers in 1 litre (2¾ pints) of boiling water, and drink two large cups before going to bed.

MANDARIN JUICE

A great alternative to tea in the hot summer months is the natural sedative mandarin, which is packed full of calming bromine.

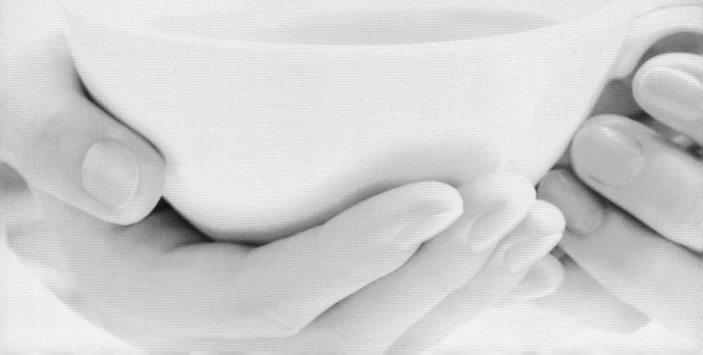

ESSENTIAL VITAMINS AND MINERALS

With our hectic daily schedules it is not always possible to eat as well as we would like to, which can leave our systems depleted of much-needed vitamins and minerals. There are ways of combating these lapses, but the most important thing to consider when buying a supplement is that each brand has a different concentration level; often buying a cheap version with too low a level will have little impact. Some also need to be taken together in order to promote absorption, and some should not be taken with food for the same reason.

Some vitamin and mineral supplements should not be taken at night as they can stimulate brain activity, especially if they contain vitamin B complex, which will erode your good night's sleep. When choosing a supplement, don't just assume that the

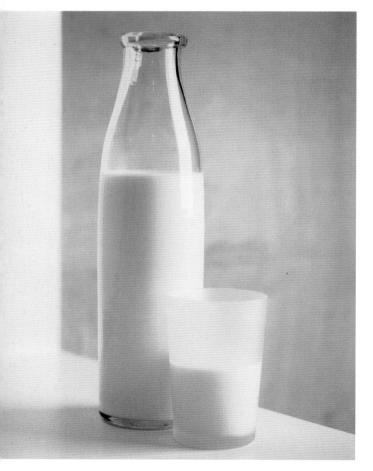

more you take, the better you will feel. Some products can be harmful when consumed in high amounts or in combination with certain other substances. If in doubt, check with your healthcare provider before taking a supplement, especially when combining them with or substituting them for other foods or medicine or if you are pregnant.

As you will see below, you can maximize your intake of several vitamins and minerals by simply increasing your intake of certain foods.

Vitamin B Complex

This helps the body to cope in times of stress; helps prevent depression and aids women who suffer from pre-menstrual syndrome, B6 specifically. It is especially effective if taken at times of extreme pressure, helping to banish feelings of helplessness and the often resulting insomnia. To be most effective, a vitamin B complex must contain thiamine, riboflavin, niacin, folate and B12.

Naturally occurring: You can boost your intake by eating poultry, green leafy vegetables, fish, nuts, seeds, wholegrain products, red meat, soya, potatoes and yeast.

Calcium

Our stressful lives often trigger the 'fight or flight' mechanism that switches on the stress hormone noradrenalin, which causes the body to excrete calcium from the bones. Calcium promotes a good night's sleep, so it needs to be replaced, especially by women, who often suffer from osteoporosis after menopause. Take calcium with magnesium and vitamin D to aid absorption.

Naturally occurring: You will find calcium in dairy products, such as milk and cheese, pulses, canned fish with bones, green leafy vegetables, soya, sesame seeds and tofu.

LEFT **Milk is an excellent source of calcium – 560 ml (1 pint) provides an adult's recommended daily allowance, as well as other essential vitamins and minerals.**

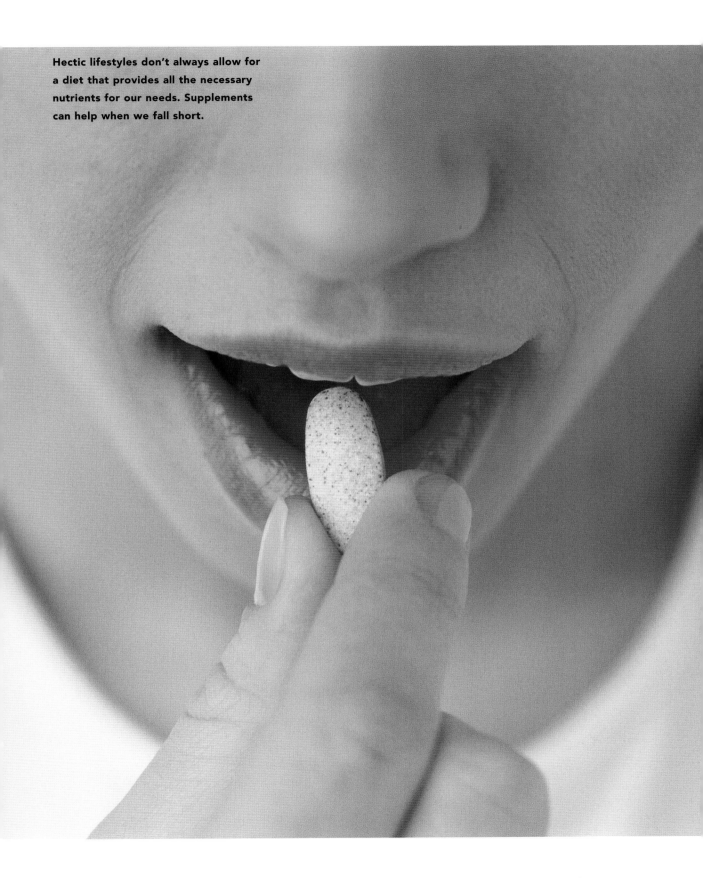

Hectic lifestyles don't always allow for a diet that provides all the necessary nutrients for our needs. Supplements can help when we fall short.

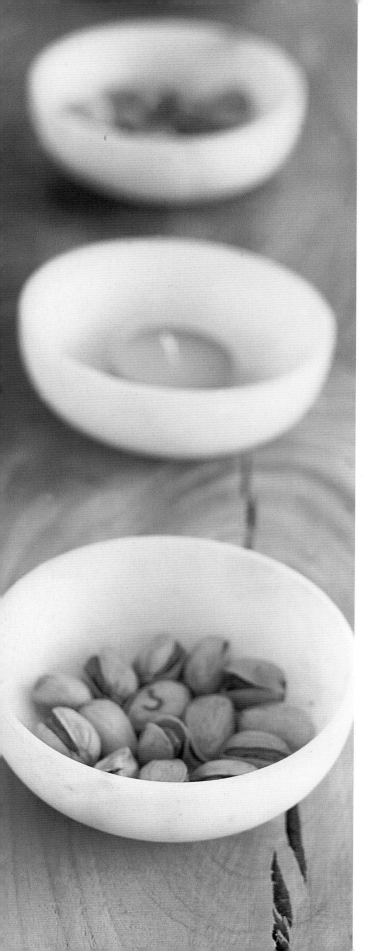

Magnesium

Magnesium is the fourth most abundant mineral in the body and is essential to good health. It is needed for more than 300 biochemical reactions and helps to maintain normal muscle and nerve function, keeps the heart rhythm steady, supports a healthy immune system and keeps bones strong. Magnesium also helps regulate blood sugar levels, promotes normal blood pressure and is known to be involved in energy metabolism.

Naturally occurring: Magnesium is found in apples, nuts, sesame seeds, figs, dried apricots, lemons and green vegetables.

Vitamin C

Like vitamin B, vitamin C is needed to turn glucose into energy. Smoking depletes it, as does alcohol, which also depletes vitamin B – this is one of the reasons you feel so awful after a night indulging in such activities. Vitamin C is an essential antioxidant that repairs the damage caused by free radicals (harmful molecules in our body) and maintains healthy skin and the operation of many of our main organs. Try not to cut vegetables and fruit into small pieces before eating them as vitamin C is oxidized by air. It is also soluble in water.

Naturally occurring: It is found in oranges and other citrus fruit, berries, strawberries, broccoli, cauliflower, raw peppers and kiwi fruit, in fact all fresh fruit and vegetables contain vitamin C.

Chromium

An essential mineral that helps stabilize appetite and prevents cravings, as well as maintaining a healthy heart. A lack of chromium can mean daytime drowsiness, cold hands, excessive thirst and an addiction to sweet foods.

LEFT **Nuts are a wonderful source of magnesium and make a healthy snack.**

RIGHT **One orange a day provides enough vitamin C for an average adult.**

Naturally occurring: It is found in wholegrain bread, brewer's yeast, oysters, potatoes, chicken, green peppers and wheatgerm.

Evening Primrose Oil

As well as its high levels of tryptophan and gamma-linolenic acid (GLA), which helps balance hormone production, this is a great aid to women suffering from sleep problems connected with premenstrual syndrome/tension (PMS/PMT) or menopause.

Kava Kava

Native to the South Pacific, the root of the kava (*Piper methysticum*) is renowned for its successful use in the overall treatment of anxiety, depression, restlessness and insomnia. Kavalactones appear to act primarily on the limbic system, the primitive part of the brain that affects all other brain activities and is the principal seat of the emotions and instinct. It is thought that kava may produce its anxiety-relieving and mood-elevating effects by altering the way in which the limbic system influences emotional processes. Unlike many preparations, it does not lead to an increased tolerance, so kava won't lose effectiveness over time. It is useful for anxiety and insomnia resulting from the menopause. For sedative effects, it should be taken one hour before you want to go to bed. Kava is restricted in many countries, and although not available in the UK or Canada, it is legal in the USA and Australia.

Melatonin

This hormone is created by a group of nerves in the brain, found just behind the eyes, called the pineal gland. Its name comes from the Greek word *melas* meaning dark or black. Melatonin is released by the pineal gland as the sun sets and makes you feel sleepy and ready for bed. It is how the body knows that it is night-time, and even what season it is. Melatonin also lowers the body temperature, which is needed to slow down the heart rate and allow the body to enter sleep mode. Sleeping in an utterly dark room increases the production of melatonin.

Clever as it is, your body cannot tell the difference between electric light and sunlight – this is one reason why we get less sleep than our ancestors. In days gone by, candles were expensive so people would spend more time in bed sleeping and in a waking state of rest. With the invention of the electric light, the hours in which we can and are expected to work and play have been extended.

Melatonin is a hormone and as such is not available for purchase in some countries, although it is available in the USA. Taking melatonin as a supplement stimulates sleep when the natural cycle is disturbed, and is particularly effective for coping with jet lag (see also page 39).

Ginseng

If your insomnia is stress related, ginseng could help you to control the attendant anxiety and protect you from stress 'burn out'. It stops you from producing excess cortisol, the stress hormone that can tip from good to bad when too much is produced and it starts to impair concentration. Ginseng keeps up the production of serotonin and norepinephrine, which guard against depression. The dip in our immune system brought on by a lack of sleep can also be corrected by ginseng, when taken in small amounts.

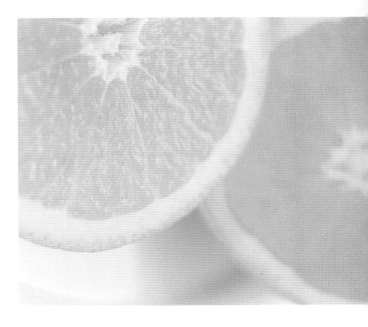

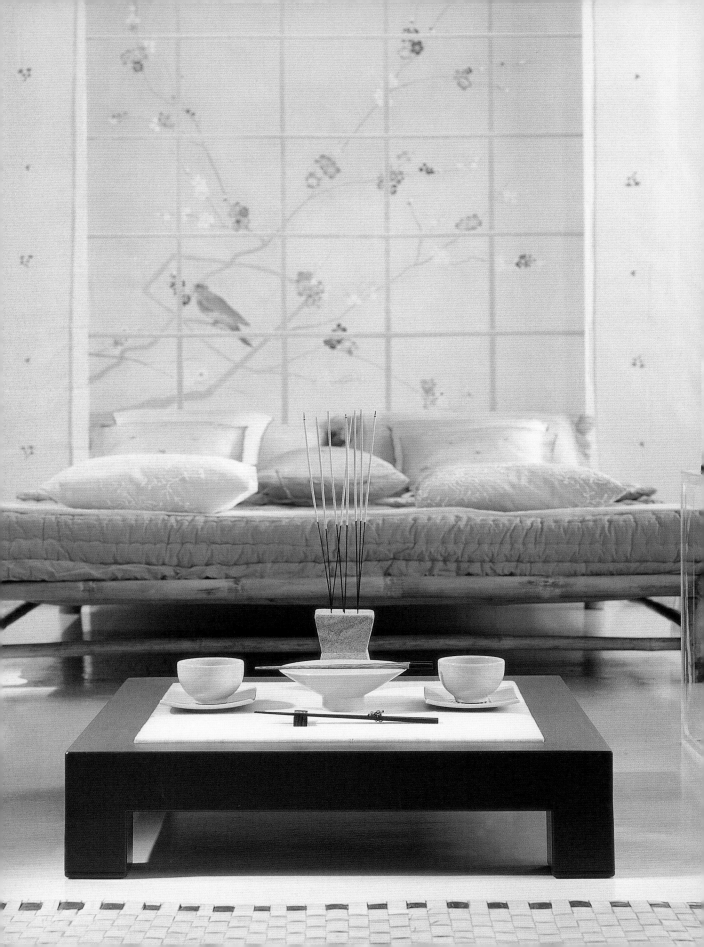

4 Creating a Sleep Haven

THE IDEA OF GOING TO BED has always been synonymous with comfort, peace and relief. Sadly, the reality is often a pale imitation of the fantasy. Many people's bedrooms are a muddle of furniture, entertainment systems, clothes and office or exercise equipment. Despite the crisis of space many of us suffer from, to ensure the best night's sleep the bedroom needs to be a retreat from all the stimulants that keep you hooked into your daytime concerns.

First, try this quick quiz to determine whether your bedroom is a sanctuary or a cell. For each yes answer score one point, for each no, zero.

• Do you take longer than 20 minutes to fall asleep?
• Do you have one light source in the bedroom?
• Do you have a TV in your bedroom?
• Is your bedroom dual purpose (e.g., an office)?
• Do you lack adequate storage in your bedroom?
• Do you sleep near a busy road or experience other forms of noise pollution?
• Do you wake feeling groggy?
• Do you ever wake up repeatedly in the night?
• Do you share a bed regularly with someone else?
• Are you reliant on tea or coffee to start the day?

Answering yes to three or more means you need to re-evaluate your sleep space. The following section will give you ideas for improvements.

LEFT **Creating a dedicated, balanced and harmonious sleep space will help you to relax after a hectic day.**

THE RIGHT EQUIPMENT

Sound a bit scientific? The reality is that you need the right conditions to get a restful night. Just a small investment can help you to reap the rewards with a more refreshing night's rest.

The Bed

The first step when carrying out a review of your sleep is to take a look at your mattress. If you are having painful or disrupted sleep, it should be your first port of call, as it could be your body's way of simply saying that you need a new bed. We move around in our sleep up to 60 times in the night, so your bed needs to give enough room to manoeuvre. If you share your bed, you need to buy the largest you can; bear in mind that a standard double gives both partners less space than a single bed each would.

A good mattress will last you ten years at best. After ten years, a bed that is used regularly will have deteriorated by as much as 75 per cent from its new condition. Considerable back pain or restlessness can be put down to your deteriorating level of support. Mattresses come with various

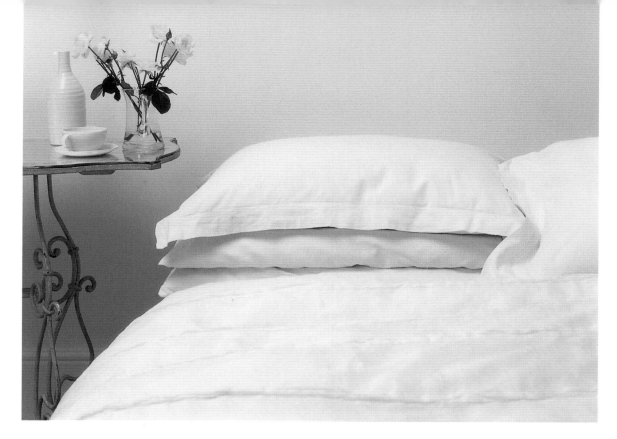

types of internal spring unit (open coil, pocket sprung or continuous springing), ordinary foam, visco-elastic or latex foam (which mould to the body) or can be filled with cotton or other fibres, or be designed to relieve particular orthopaedic difficulties. In general, the higher the spring count in a mattress, the better the support. As a guide, the higher the spring count, the more you will pay.

A divan bed has springs in the base as well as the mattress that are designed to work together. If you have a more basic bed frame, without springs, make sure you buy a good mattress to compensate for the lack of support in the base. A myth that persists is that the firmer the mattress, the better it is for your back. The level of firmness should actually relate to your body weight – the heavier you are, the firmer your bed needs to be. The mattress should allow your 'sticking-out bits' – your hips and shoulders – to press into the mattress so that your 'sticking-in bits' – your waist or the small of your back – is supported. If you have a specific joint or back problem, take advice from an osteopath or healthcare professional who will be able to advise you.

ABOVE **A good mattress deserves a suitable amount of investment as it is essential for providing support and comfort for the resting body.**

Make sure you test lots of mattresses as they vary massively from one manufacturer to another. If you share your bed with someone, make sure they try it too, in order to ensure you both have enough room and don't roll together. If you can't compromise, then look at zip and link beds, which join two single beds together. These have welcome advantages for those who have widely differing comfort and support requirements.

When buying your bed there is still one last element to consider – to store or not to store. A lack of storage in the bedroom can be simply solved by purchasing a bed base with drawers underneath, but bear in mind that these are not as good for your back as a sprung base. In some cases, however, losing a degree of comfort more than makes up for getting rid of the piles of boxes or clothes that distract you from rest.

Pillows

Good-quality pillows are vital in the fight against neck and back pain. Choose a mix of duck down for comfort and feathers for support. If you suffer from a feather allergy, there are good synthetic versions, although they won't last as long so be aware that they will need replacing sooner. As with duvets, pillows should be cleaned regularly every four to six months. Feather pillows can be dry cleaned, hand washed or machine washed. Make sure there are no holes in the casing, then wash on a cool wash with a mild detergent. Afterwards, dry on a hot setting in your tumble dryer or hang out in the sun; whichever method you choose, make sure the pillows are thoroughly dry. Placed in a pillowcase, a damp pillow will get mildew and be ruined. For those with dust allergies, pillows that can be regularly laundered in the washing machine are ideal.

If you tend to wake up with a sore neck, then it could be down to the positioning of your pillows. As you enter REM sleep, your muscles are relaxed and only the ligaments are holding your head in place. Your head, therefore, needs to be held in a straight line with your body; not bent towards the bed toward your chest when you are flat on your back. Experiment with one or two pillows to see what works best for you.

Duvets

The common choice for bedding these days is a duvet or comforter, so when selecting one you need to understand the 'tog' rating that is usually applied to them. Tog is a measurement of warmth: the higher the tog, the warmer the duvet. A child should be fine with a 4.5 tog duvet all year round in mild climates, but in winter an adult may need a duvet with a rating of between 12 and 13.5. A good way to match the rating with the season is to buy a low-tog spring duvet, about 4 togs, and a heavier one, about 9 togs, and combine them in the winter. Women get colder in bed at night than men, so they may need a higher tog. There are now duvets with a separate tog rating on each side to allow for couples with different preferences.

Sheets

Choice of sheets is a case of personal preference, but linen is kindest on the skin as it is natural and PH neutral. It can absorb up to 20 per cent of its own weight in moisture, thus absorbing some of the 280 ml (½ pint) of water we lose every night in perspiration. The higher the thread count, the finer the weave and the softer it will feel on the skin. Although linen is more expensive than cotton, it will last for many years so will be a good investment. If cotton is your preference, apply the same thread count rule as per linen for softness; anything with fewer than 180 will feel rough on the skin.

BELOW **Whether you prefer linen or cotton, for good-quality sheets the general rule is the higher the thread count, the softer the sheet.**

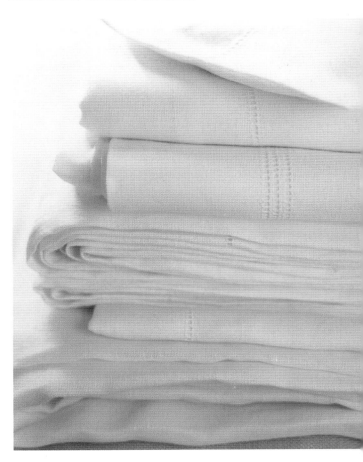

Nightwear

Unless you like to sleep as nature intended, wear nightwear that is made of natural fibres to help the skin to breathe and cope with fluctuating body and external temperatures. The clothing should be soft, warm and comfortable. Ensure you don't choose items that are too tight or likely to get caught up in the bedding.

Bed socks work for those who suffer from chilly extremities, and can even comfort and aid restless sleepers with no temperature problems. By keeping the extremities warm and thus making you more comfortable, bed socks allow the core body temperature to drop further, which promotes deeper relaxation – intense relaxation through meditation has also been shown to lower the body temperature.

Allergies

Some allergy sufferers can find that bedtime exacerbates their symptoms, causing them to lie awake trying to catch their breath and sneezing. To help keep dust and dust mites to a minimum, vacuum and launder bedding frequently, use hypoallergenic pillows and bedding and keep pets out of the bedroom. As well as the bed, take a good look around your room for possible triggers – padded bed heads, carpets and cushions can all harbour dust and mites. One very common misconception is that feathers should be avoided, as people often think that feathers irritate all allergies – in fact, they only affect those with a feather allergy! Natural bedding is often a good option for allergy sufferers as it is usually enclosed in a tighter woven casing, so is pretty dust-mite-proof. If you are unsure about the cause of your problems, ask your doctor about being tested.

RIGHT **There is more to allergy-proofing a room than avoiding feather pillows. Fabric-covered bed heads, curtains and carpets also need special treatment.**

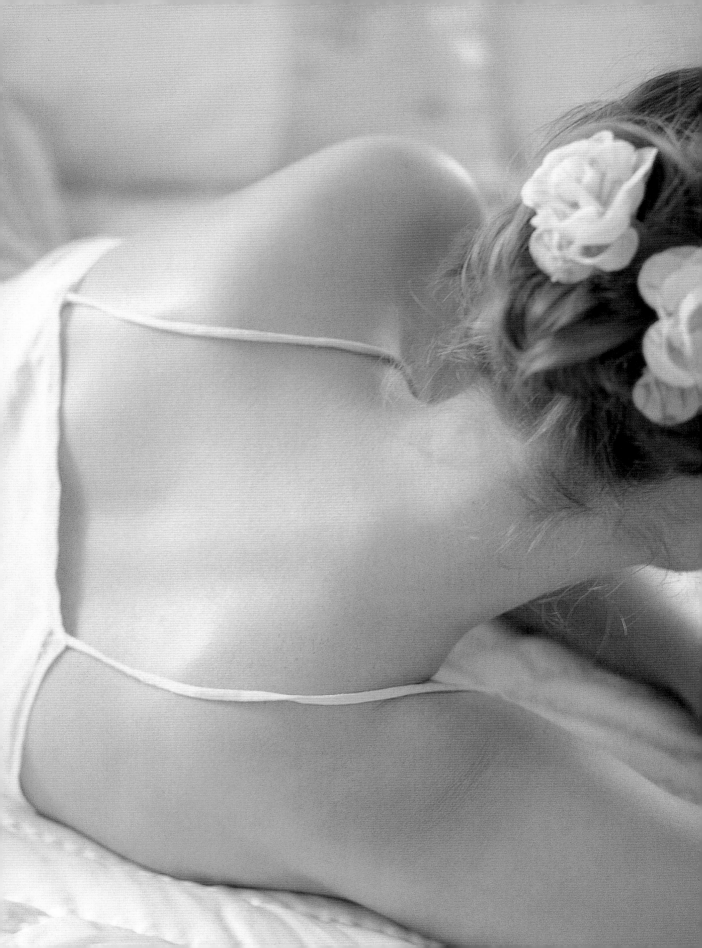

AMBIENCE

Now that you have all the equipment in place, it is time to consider the ambience of your sleep space. We are especially sensitive to our environment when entering the first stage of sleep, as we can be easily disturbed (see page 12), and it is essential that we feel relaxed, comfortable and safe in order to go to sleep. Here are some ways you can improve the environment you sleep in.

Lighting

Most importantly, you need to get the room lighting correct. For the body to activate the 'go to sleep' hormone melatonin, it needs darkness. Gentle, low lighting in the bedroom, therefore, allows the body slowly to prepare for sleep. With this in mind, choose low-level lamps that give off a diffused light; this also has the advantage of creating a relaxing, intimate mood.

Architects and designers call this kind of gentle lighting 'mood lighting', but because in winter months you also need your bedroom lighting to be bright enough to allow you to dress and prepare for the day, you will need brighter 'task lighting' – your lighting plan should allow for both. Fitting a dimmer switch to the overhead light will give you the most range. If you share a bedroom, bedside lamps are invaluable for allowing one person to read and the other to snooze. The ultimate luxury is a switch by both the bed and the door, or even

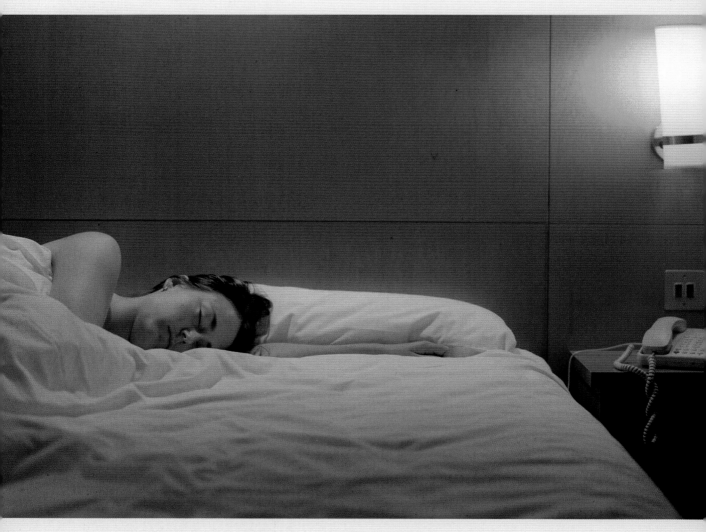

voice-activated ones, so that you don't even have to get out of bed to turn off the lights. When tackling children's rooms, low-level lighting, such as a night-light, means you can leave it switched on without disturbing the child's sleep. Dimmer switches can also be used to help your child recognize that bedtime is approaching.

The light as you wake is just as important as the light when you are trying to sleep. While it is necessary to keep strong light, such as irritating street lights, out of the room to allow you to nod off, you also need to make sure there is enough light coming in to let the body know when to start rousing you from your slumber. A window treatment that shuts out the emerging dawn will encourage the production of extra melatonin, which will lead to a drugged and disorientated sensation upon waking up. Thick, heavy curtains will keep you warmer in winter, but will also produce this effect. If you have no other choice but to opt for total blackout, buy a light-activated alarm clock that imitates the onset of dawn and helps the body prepare for waking up by releasing the 'wake up' hormone cortisol. To allow natural light to wake you, try diffusing it with voile or muslin curtains.

A good tip is to treat yourself to a visit to a sumptuous hotel to see how the experts create appealing sleep spaces. Perhaps steal a few ideas, such as bedside lamps mounted on the wall or downlighters – you can always justify it as research!

Temperature and Humidity

Key to a really good night's sleep is the correct temperature. The body needs to cool down to allow the core temperature of the internal organs, like the heart and lungs, to slow their rate. This is why hot summer nights can make it so difficult to sleep. Cool – not cold – conditions are the best for

LEFT **Gentle lighting is essential for creating a calming mood in the bedroom and for letting the body (and an active mind) know that it is time to rest.**

good sleep and the ideal temperature should be between 16–18°C (60–65°F). Even on chilly winter nights, when it might be tempting to turn up the heating, you should try to maintain this level. If you are cold, don't just throw a heavy blanket over the bed to keep you warm, as this can affect the efficiency of the duvet. Instead, replace your duvet or team it with another one for a heavier tog value. Alternatively, put the blanket under the duvet or buy a thin electric blanket.

Humidity is also an essential element for good sleep. Central heating can dry the air in living spaces and make breathing become difficult or uncomfortable. If you wake up with a sore throat or dryness in your nose, the room probably has too little humidity. You may be unable to sleep with the window open, because of pollution or noise, but humidifiers, which release moisture into the air, can prevent the room from seeming dry and stuffy. You can achieve a similar effect by placing a bowl of water near the radiator or heater in your room.

Blocking Out Noise

Noise is not always such a bad thing. Although it would be wonderful to sleep in total silence, sharing a planet with lots of other people means this is frequently unachievable. People often wake up, roused by noise, as they enter the lighter part of their sleep cycle – this is often more a problem for older people who spend less time in deep sleep and more in the kind that is easily disturbed by noise. You can, of course, use sound insulation if you live on a busy road, such as double glazing, insulation between floors and walls, or choose a room in the quietest spot of the house away from main roads or good old-fashioned ear plugs. However, an effective trick can be to add some noise of your own. The low-level whir of a fan can often block out distracting noises, and once you have become used to the sound, you may find that it no longer disturbs you at all. If you have ever fallen asleep in front of a flickering TV, the effect of a comforting low-level background noise will be familiar.

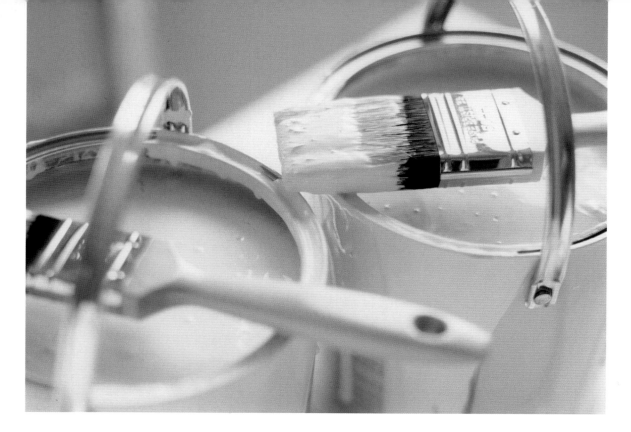

Colour Yourself Sleepy

Colour has an incredibly far-reaching effect on our emotions; for example, orange is known to stimulate mental activity and red represents power, drive, action and passion. When choosing a colour for your bedroom, therefore, it is not always wise to go with your favourite colour. If you have a colour that you really want to use, like purple, try a paler version of it such as lilac; it will be much more restful. You can then use it in its bolder form as accents such as cushions or throws.

The most reflective colours are associated with calm in nature: dusky pinks of late summer skies, soft greens of pastures, pale blues of wildflowers. Other colours can be used in more intense shades and still feel restful, such as turquoise and pink.

In conjunction with the Colour and Imaging Institute at the University of Derby in the UK, Angela Wright created a software system that analyzes the most appropriate use of colour based on emotional and psychological principles. In their pure form, the following colours are most suitable for a bedroom environment. The key to choosing a colour that creates calm rather than coldness, for

ABOVE **Colour affects us in ways that we rarely consciously acknowledge. Ensure you choose the correct colours to create a restful haven.**

example, is selecting the right shade; look at several samples and choose the one that draws you to it when you think of a calming, rather than cold space. A 'warm' shade (such as a white with a yellow undertone rather than a blue undertone) will always seem friendlier (and less like an old-fashioned hospital ward).

Blue: Essentially soothing, blue affects us mentally, calming the mind and aiding concentration. A strong blue will stimulate clear thought. Too much, or the wrong shade, can be cold.

Violet/Purple: This colour has the shortest wavelength, making it nearest to ultraviolet, and lending it mystical qualities. It encourages spiritual contemplation, and has associations with luxury, truth and awareness. Too much can cause introversion and a sense of suppression.

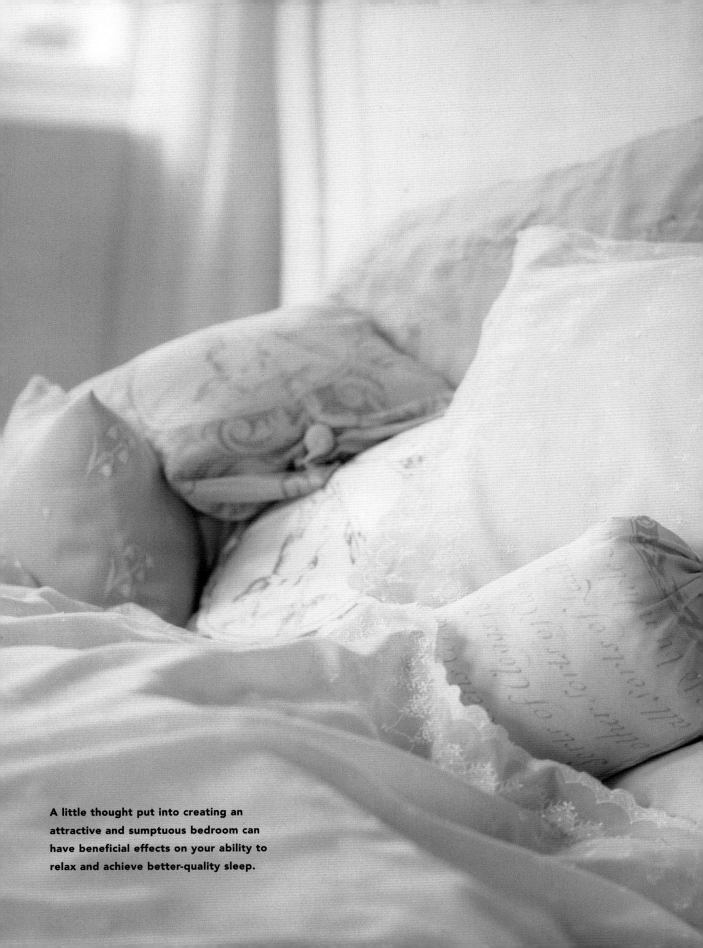

A little thought put into creating an attractive and sumptuous bedroom can have beneficial effects on your ability to relax and achieve better-quality sleep.

Pink: A physically nurturing colour, pink evokes feelings of tranquillity, warmth and love are all represented by pink, which is also the colour of femininity. It is physically soothing, but can be draining if used to excess.

Green: This colour is at the very centre of the colour spectrum, and therefore represents balance. It suggests harmony, refreshment, peace and rest. Too much can indicate stagnation or boredom.

BELOW **A monochrome scheme is restful on the eye. When using white, achieve a more interesting look and feel by using it with different textures in the bedroom.**

White: White creates a heightened perception of space, and represents purity, clarity, sophistication and simplicity. However, when used with warm colours it can make them seem garish, so accessorize carefully. White used in the wrong shade (there are many 'whites') can seem cold and unfriendly, so choose a yellow-based shade. The colour works well with texture to soften its hard implications.

Brown: Warm and soft but serious, brown communicates earth and nature. A useful neutral, it is quietly supportive in interior design. Too much can look heavy, so is best used as an accent, such as a dark wooden floor in a white room, which will help achieve softness.

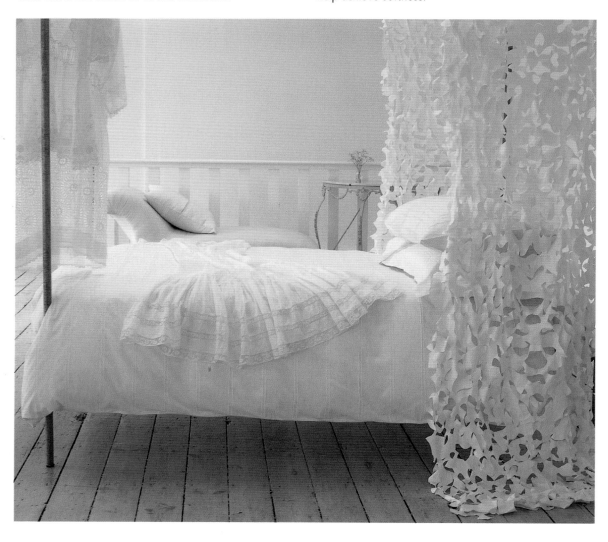

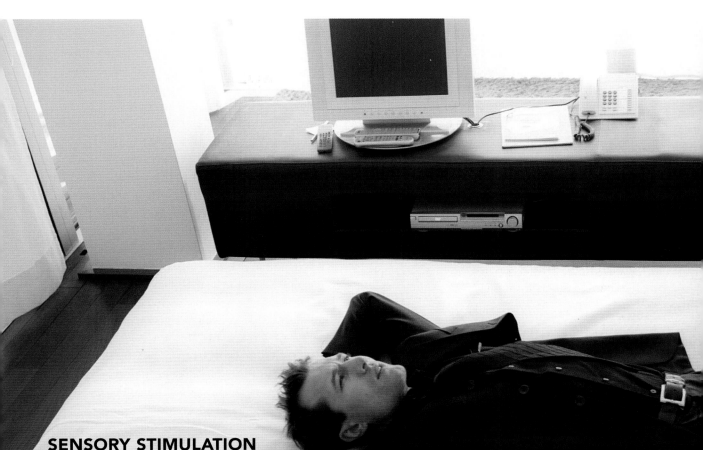

SENSORY STIMULATION

Keeping outside influences, and reminders of the active daytime world, from creeping into your sleeping environment will go far to aid rest and relaxation. There are also ways you can create sense experiences that induce sleep, from introducing comfortable fabrics to using relaxing aromas to scent the bedding and air – which can form a welcome contrast to the rest of your home and help coax the body into a state of deep relaxation.

Electronic Equipment

Two-thirds of British children have a computer, games machine or TV in their bedroom, which could mean they are losing sleep as a result. The adult population is no better. As well as encouraging you to stay up past your bedtime to send just one last email, the red 'stand-by' lights can impair your sleep quality by affecting the brain's ability to switch off. Electronic equipment needs to be moved from your sleeping space if you are to get a good night's sleep. If space is at a premium, however, and you have to work from your bedroom, use a storage system that you can fold away or, at the very least, use black tape to cover the red stand-by indicators.

ABOVE **Bedrooms often double up as places to watch TV or as home offices, which keep the mind active long after it should be winding down for sleep.**

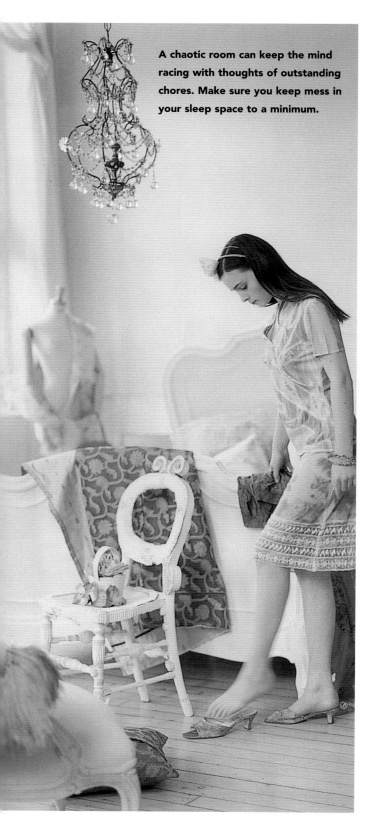

A chaotic room can keep the mind racing with thoughts of outstanding chores. Make sure you keep mess in your sleep space to a minimum.

Clear Up the Clutter

There are other distractions that should also have a veil drawn discreetly over them. Open storage might seem like an efficient way to grab a cardigan before work, but being able to see a mess out of the corner of your eye is enough to keep you wide awake just thinking about clearing it up. A clear demarcation of space is needed. Doors, or even muslin drapes, can help you to shut out mess and muddle and to switch off. Think of clutter as intellectual noise. If you leave things heaped about the room, you are doing the equivalent to your brain as inviting a brass band to play while you try to sleep. Even if you are too tired to tidy that night, throw everything into a basket and put it outside the bedroom door. You can deal with it tomorrow when you are more refreshed.

Introduce Texture

Texture is essential for bringing interest and comfort to a bedroom. A neutral relaxing colour scheme, such as a mixture of off-whites and camel colours, can be given extra depth and interest by throwing a woven blanket over the foot of the bed, or hanging some heavy, chunky cord curtains. Don't just opt for one type of texture. If you would like some personal mementos to keep the theme fun and sleep-inspiring, a collection of black-and-white photographs of loved ones is stylish without making you forget why you are there.

You can also use texture to try something new. If you are getting over a sleep problem, or just want to shake off old associations, try a gauzy canopy over the bed, a string of tiny lights around the bed head instead of a reading lamp, or a dramatic window treatment; choose a focal point and make the most of it.

RIGHT **Texture can add much-needed interest to a room. If accessories are taken from a palate of similar tones, the overall effect remains calming and neutral.**

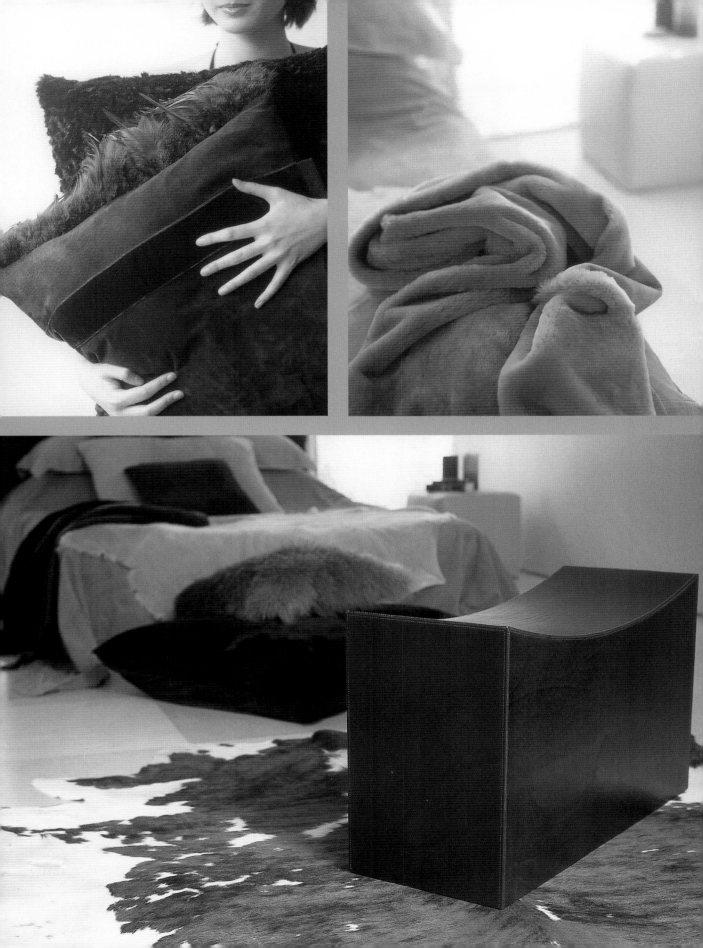

Pep Up the Passion

Use music and scent to quickly change the energy in your bedroom after a long, demanding day. Choose something sultry, rather than distracting, for background noise (yes to easy jazz, no to heavy rock, unless you want your partner to break off to do a guitar solo halfway through). Scent acts very quickly to alter an atmosphere: try ylang ylang in an oil burner, as the flickering light will also enhance the mood. A row of candles standing on a long mirror will also add a sense of occasion. If your partner still can't shake off the stress of the day, get them to try this simple 'state breaker', which will instantly encourage them to release themselves from their mood. Sit straight with your eyes closed, then breathe in deeply through the nose and out slowly through the mouth; repeat three times to attain a more relaxed state.

BELOW **The bedroom is more than just a place to sleep. By using lighting, scent and music you can change the mood to one for getting in the mood.**

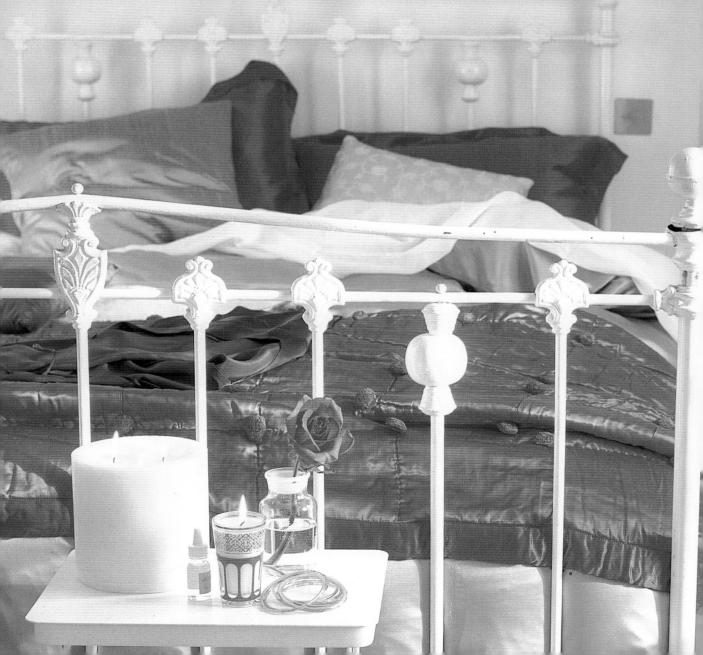

SLEEP RITUALS

Bedtime rituals are known to help children to prepare for a good night's sleep. The repetition of the same routine gradually unwinds the mind and body and indicates to them that nearing bedtime can be wonderfully soothing and achieve effective results. It's obvious, but easy to forget, that creating a slightly more sophisticated version can have the same success for adults.

A Bathroom Retreat

One of the most effective routines is to have a nightly bath. The calming properties of water have clear effects on our senses and can be used to refresh and revive, or improve, our mood and calm us. Creating different atmospheres in your bathroom will help achieve both ends, and using different fragrances will enhance the effect.

A warm, but not too hot, bath works by increasing the body temperature, which then begins to drop, mimicking the body's reaction to the onset of sleep. For many of us who share a home, have a chaotic work schedule or even work from home, it is a great way to change the pace of your day by signifying some time specifically for yourself and your relaxation needs. Even preparing your bathroom for your soak can be restful. Research has shown that low-level tasks, such as cleaning or organizing, can help balance the mind and relieve stress. If you repeat the same process nightly, you will start to relax as soon as you hang your towel on the radiator.

First, you need to eliminate all the unnecessary clutter in your bathroom. This may seem difficult as many bathrooms tend to be small, but there is room for improvement in most situations so invest in some stacking boxes that won't take up much floor space, and pack away children's toys or the products you don't use every day but would like to keep. Before you simply put things away, though, ask yourself when was the last time you used them – a lot of perfumed products go 'off', so as a rule if you haven't used something in two months you should use it up quickly or throw it away. Replace

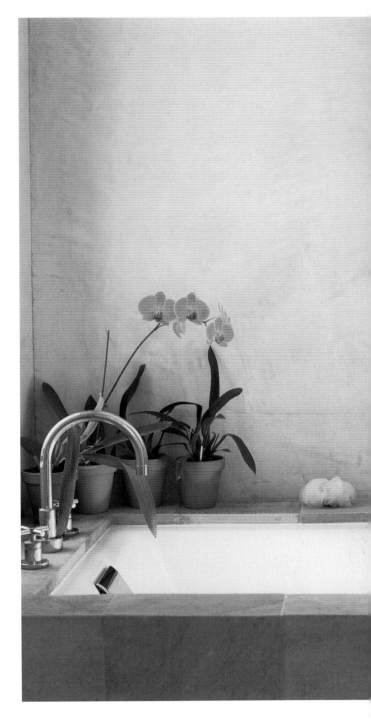

ABOVE **Almost any bathroom can be turned into a mini spa retreat with clever storage, plants, evocative scents and lighting. A lock on the door can also keep the rest of the world at bay.**

open shelves, if you aren't disciplined enough to keep them tidy, with slim cupboards with doors. If you don't want to get shampoo or conditioner from the cupboard every day, swap half-empty, sticky bottles for more aesthetically pleasing pump-dispenser containers that go with your colour scheme. Getting rid of a multicoloured chaos of plastic junk will immediately make a space more calming. Don't forget to look up – a shelf above a door utilizes often 'dead' space and can be used to house clutter-containing baskets or rolled up towels; you could even put your homemade relaxation kit up there, out of the way of small prying hands.

Once de-cluttered, you should put together a kit designed especially for you. A sumptuous bath sheet to wrap yourself in when you emerge is essential, but try not to use fabric softener on your towels as it coats the fibres with a substance that tends to stiffen them.

Candles that contain aromatherapy oils, or oils in an oil burner, will provide a soothing, flickering, melatonin-triggering low light and a calming fragrance. Finally, include something scented in your bath to promote rest. As you become accustomed to your ritual, the evocative nature of scent, which is known to generate memory recall, will make you associate this daily routine with calm and peace. Try one of these relaxing, stress-balancing recipes:

- The colour and pretty daisylike shape of camomile flowers are lovely to look at; sprinkle the heads into the bath and sip a cup of camomile tea while soaking.

- A combination of Dead Sea salts with a few drops of sandalwood and lavender essential oils will rest both aching muscles and a tired mind. For a choice of other calming scents and their properties, see pages 93–7 on aromatherapy.

Before you go into the bathroom, deal with annoying stresses so that you don't lie there fretting. Put the washing machine on, have

LEFT **Treat yourself to some huge, soft bath towels so that you can feel warm and safe after a mood-changing and restful bath.**

RIGHT **The scent of flowers, such as rose and camomile, can help ease away anxiety and worries. Use them in their flower or petal form as a visual treat, too.**

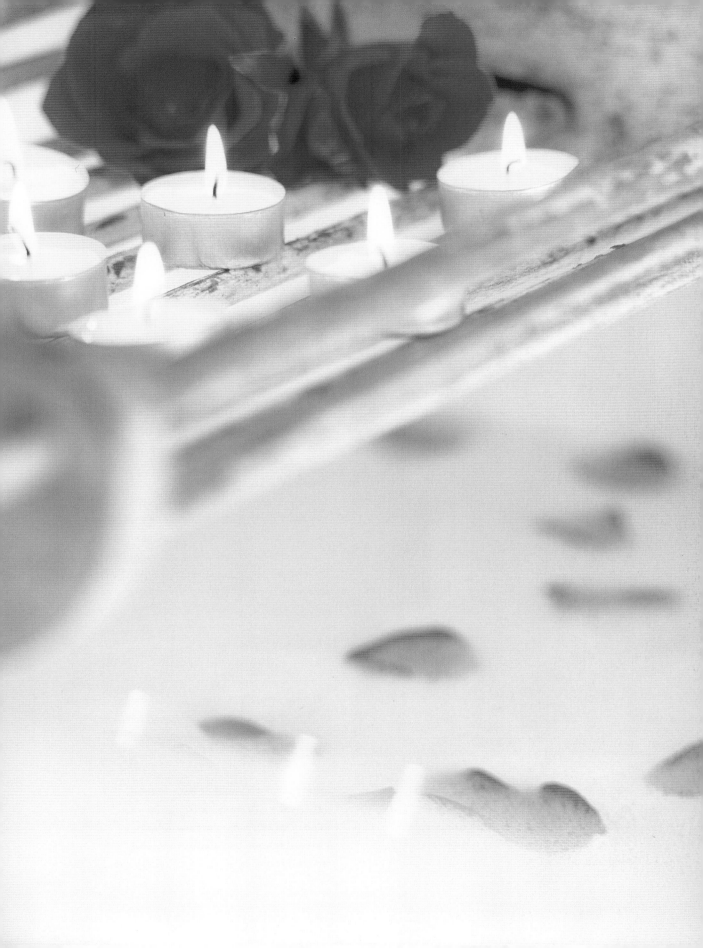

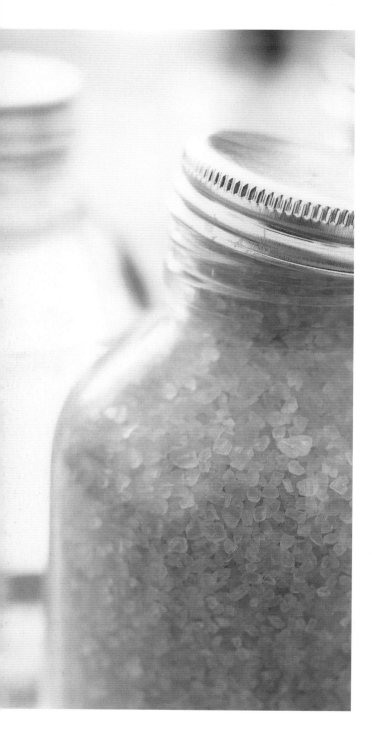

any chats about the day's demands with those who need filling in, then make it clear that you are not available for the next 30 minutes. You may even want to hang a 'Do Not Disturb' sign on the door; someone knocking to ask if you've paid the phone bill can be very disruptive.

Bathtime might be the time to get out your notepad. Write down any of the stresses that have happened during the day, errands you feel you need to deal with, or things that worry you. Writing them down will help you put them aside while you sleep, and sleeping well will allow you to cope with them much better the following day. You will often find that half of the things you are worrying about don't actually need any attention; they are just the product of an overwrought mind. If you don't want to write them down in the bath, keeping a notepad by the bed is also a good way of 'doing' something about worries that may cause insomnia. You also need to grant yourself 'permission' to go to bed, and not feel that you are shirking responsibilities.

Self Massage

While you are warm, clean and peaceful, it is a great time to perform some self-massage techniques. You can make your own massage oil, but be careful to avoid using stimulating blends by mistake or just because they are the only ones you have to hand. Try this aromatherapy blend to encourage the onset of slumber:

4 drops of lavender
3 drops of camomile
3 drops of clary sage
Carrier oil such as olive, sunflower or almond oil (25 ml/1 fl oz of carrier oil should have only 12–15 drops of essential oil added).

ABOVE **Put together a kit of your most effective and relaxing aromatherapy or bath-oil scents. Reach for this emotional first aid kit whenever a day has been long and difficult.**

RIGHT **Making a ritual of your bathing experience will create a trigger in your mind. This will help start the relaxing process as soon as you head towards the bathroom.**

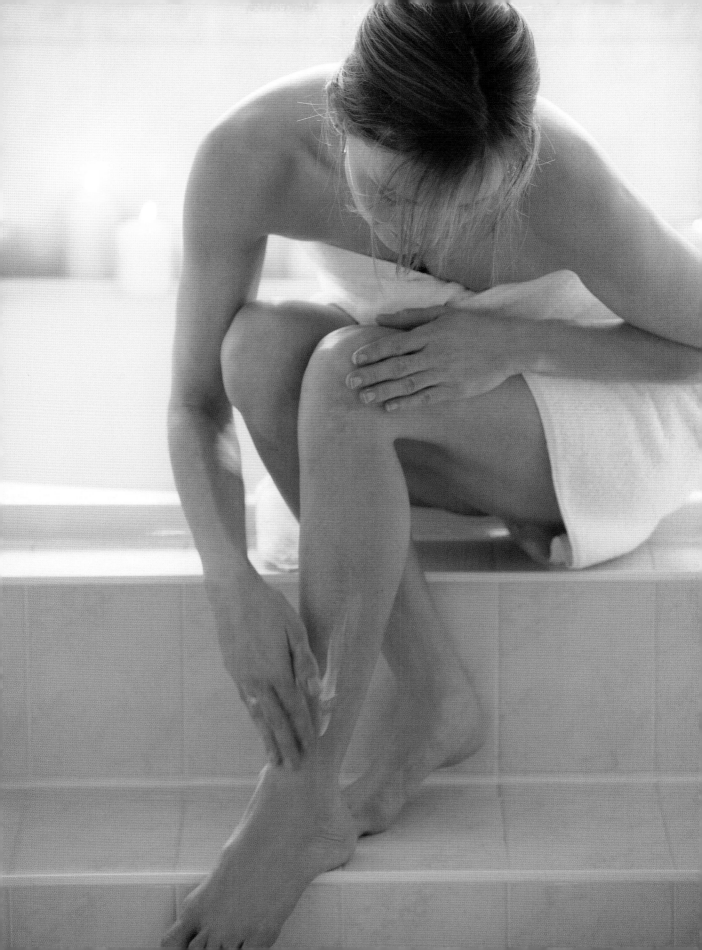

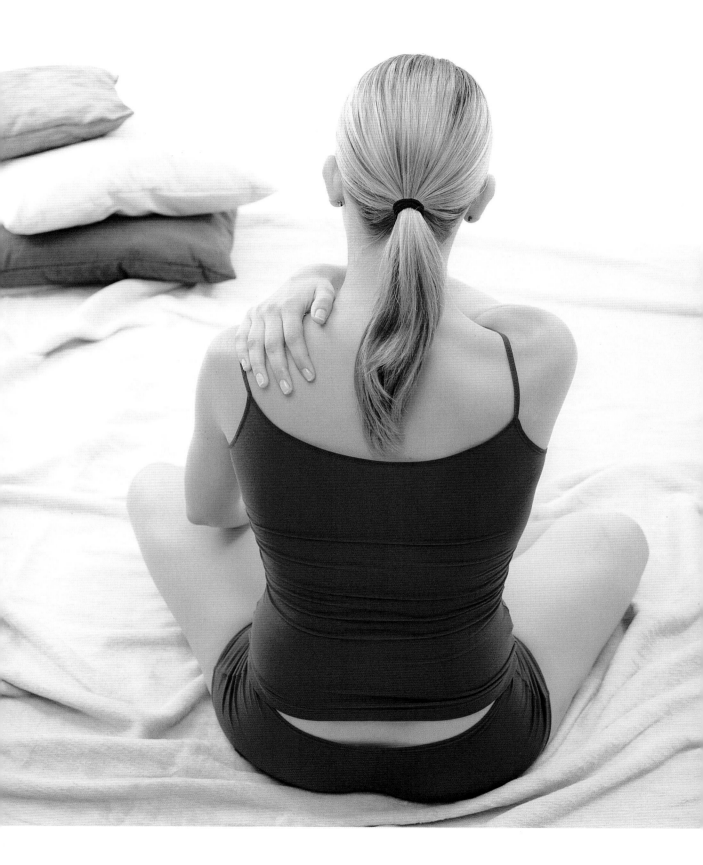

SHOULDERS

Our shoulders are often the area that holds the most stress and tension, especially if we spend the day hunched over a desk. You may want to sit in a comfy chair or on the floor for the following two massages. For the first massage, use the first two fingers of each hand.

1 Begin by placing them in the hollow just inside your collarbone, at the base of your neck – you will know when you have hit the right spot, and you will feel the tension. Press gently once, and release.

2 Repeat the pressing action along the shoulders, outwards and towards the shoulder joint.

3 Repeat the whole process five times, then change hands and work on the other shoulder.

For the next shoulder massage, you will start by using the middle three fingers of your right hand to work on the left shoulder, and then switch sides.

1 Use a firm pressure here, not enough to feel painful, but enough to release the build-up of tension.

2 Find the large triangular-shaped muscle where a lot of tension is stored, just below the shoulder.

3 Starting from the outer edge of the shoulder and working towards the spine, use your fingers to massage in a circular motion.

4 Repeat for as long as you need to, before using the same technique, with the left hand, on the other side.

LEFT **Self-massage techniques are easy to learn and can provide comfort for a tired body. Invest in some massage tools to help you to achieve the feeling of having had a professional spa massage.**

HANDS

A great deal of stress and tension can be held in the hands. This technique is especially beneficial if you use a computer as part of your everyday routine. Your thumb and index finger will do the work here. Start with your right hand working on the left, and then switch over.

1 Make a gentle pinching movement along each finger in turn, starting at the base and moving along towards the fingertip.

2 Repeat three times on each hand, before returning to the left palm.

3 Loosen the palm with your right thumb, working in a circular motion. Repeat with your other hand.

4 Return again to your left hand, loosening the back with your three middle right-hand fingers and working from the base of the fingers to the wrist. Repeat on the other hand.

FEET

They carry us around all day, but feet are often neglected. A simple foot massage can relieve tension and ease aches. A foot massage benefits the whole body, stimulating the many thousands of nerve endings there.

1 Use a little foot cream or olive oil to nourish the foot as you work.

2 Hold your feet with your thumbs facing inwards towards the sole, and gradually work around it, kneading firmly but gently.

3 Rub in small circular motions on the sole, then work on the upper part of the foot. For a great boost to circulation, carry on working up the calf, towards the heart, in gentle pressing motions.

4 Press the inside back of the ankle (the slight hollow) with the thumb to promote circulation further.

RELAXATION METHODS

Learning to relax effectively, and when you want to, should have a dramatic effect on your ability to go to sleep, stay asleep and generally get more from your waking hours. After activating our stress responses, we need effective ways to rebalance; this is where relaxation exercises like meditation, muscle relaxation and yoga can help. Here are some very immediate ideas that you can try when you are lying in your bed. First, prepare your environment to ensure it is conducive to relaxation. The checklist below may be helpful when setting the scene.

• When you are relaxed your body temperature drops, so make sure the room is warm enough to accommodate this change, but not too stuffy.

• Dress in your sleepwear, and then you won't have to disrupt your mood by changing before bed.

• Use a 'Do Not Disturb' sign to ensure peace and quiet; you may also want to put on low music to drown out background noise.

Meditation

As well as unwinding tight muscles, which can mean an uncomfortable and unrefreshing rest, meditation can calm an anxious mind and keep us from lying awake until the small hours fretting needlessly over small worries.

The classic image is of someone sitting cross-legged with their eyes closed, quietly chanting. This, of course, is just one way of approaching meditation. If you are pressured for time and feel pulled in several directions, the mere thought of meditation may seem impossible, so give yourself permission to take time out from your stressful environment. Sit in a quiet space, on a straightback chair (the support will help open up the lungs), and place a hand on your stomach. Consciously try to fill your lungs with slow, long breaths, in through your nose and out through your mouth. It may take a little practice, but you will know it is working if you feel your stomach rise and fall under your hand. Repeat this until you feel calm again. Once you have mastered the practice, you can use it anywhere – in your own living room or even in the office.

Meditation and visualization can transport you to a place that is peaceful and serene, leading you toward a relaxed state of mind.

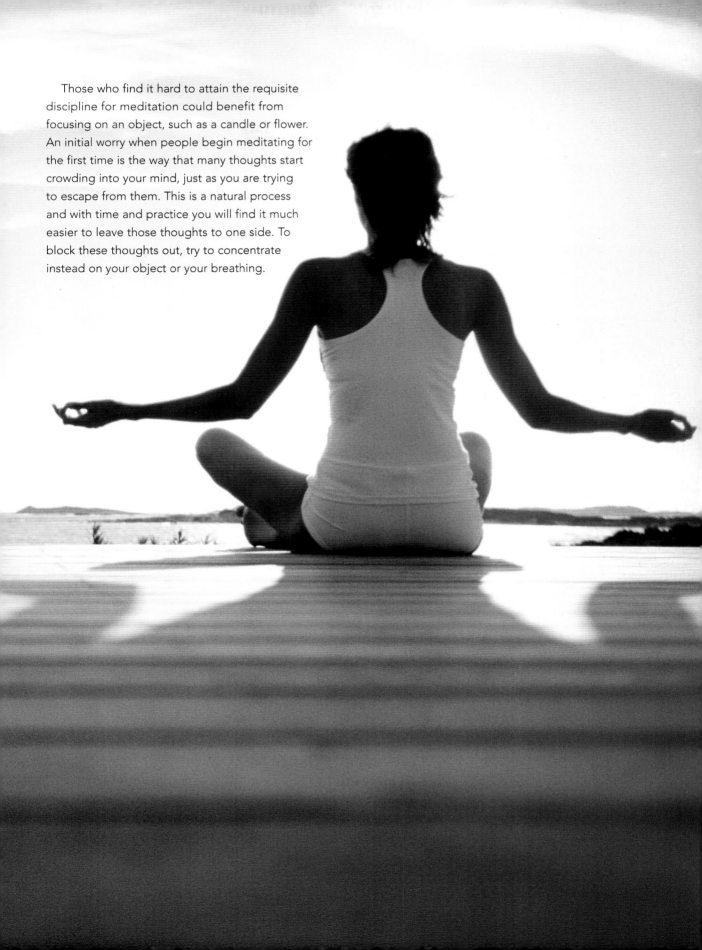

Those who find it hard to attain the requisite discipline for meditation could benefit from focusing on an object, such as a candle or flower. An initial worry when people begin meditating for the first time is the way that many thoughts start crowding into your mind, just as you are trying to escape from them. This is a natural process and with time and practice you will find it much easier to leave those thoughts to one side. To block these thoughts out, try to concentrate instead on your object or your breathing.

Breathing

Sometimes, no matter how much you need it, sleep just won't seem to come. Learning simple breathing exercises can help. In yoga this is called diaphragmatic breathing, and is profoundly relaxing. Using your abdomen, not your chest, breathe through your nose for three seconds, then breathe out through your mouth for three seconds. Pause for three seconds before repeating. Practise for ten minutes each night and you may find that you don't remember doing the last few exercises!

Research has shown that imagining a place of calm, like a favourite holiday destination, can also help speed the onset of sleep – it has even been shown to be more effective than counting sheep. This method, called creative visualization, is a very simple process to learn. Lie in your bed (try the 'Corpse' yoga position on page 84) and visualize a serene place. Imagine all the sensations that come with this place – the warmth of the sun on your skin, the babbling sound of a mountain stream and even the sweet scent of the grass. This process can be used in conjunction with progressive muscular relaxation (see below). Once relaxed, you can start focusing on your breathing, and imagining the stresses and tensions of your muscles, as a colour or sensation, leaving your body as you breathe out.

Progressive Muscular Relaxation

This systematic relaxation of the muscle groups is a useful technique for anyone who finds themselves tense and agitated at the end of the day. It is a widely acknowledged fact that anxiety, stress, depression and emotional distress can all cause muscle fatigue and tightness. Working on these muscle groups and releasing contractions can therefore help ease the problems that put the tension there in the first place. A physiologist called Dr Jacobson devised PMR to achieve this state of relaxation.

Concentrate on tightening a specific group of muscles, hold the contraction and then slowly release the tension, breathing out, with a sigh

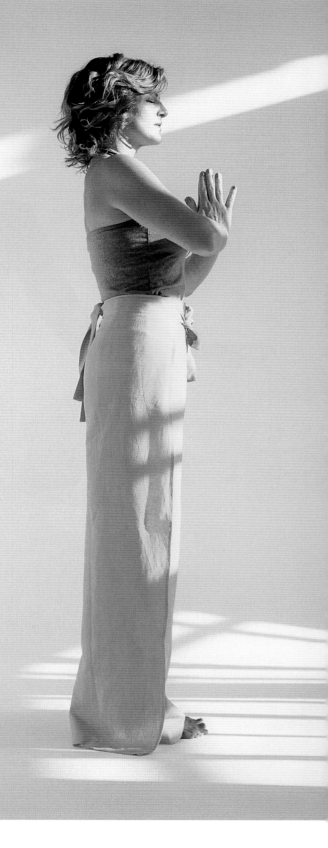

through the mouth as the tension ebbs away. Visualizing this outward flow of stressful energy will enhance the effect. Repeat on various other muscle groups. As with any form of relaxation, the effectiveness of the technique and your sensitivity to it will improve with practise and you will soon be able to relax at will.

Yoga

Designed to unify the body and mind, yoga promotes strength, good health and inner peace. It has many separate disciplines and can be invaluable in combating insomnia – even a beginner can reap the benefits. Central to effective yoga practice is learning to understand and gain control of your breathing. This can be of great help, even when we don't combine it with the specific poses. Breathing helps us to calm anxieties and clear our mind when we find ourselves under pressure.

Although there are many yoga books and videos available, it is useful to attend a class while you are getting to grips with the basics. Once these basics are mastered, you can then do them pretty much wherever you like. If practised regularly, stamina, flexibility, muscle tone, strength and energy levels will all improve. The ability to calm the mind, enter a relaxed state and improve your mood and sense of well-being will also be in your grasp.

Choosing the right class and exploring new forms are vital for anyone hoping to get the most from yoga. The main types are explained below.

• Hatha yoga is the most accessible type for a beginner to take up and you will find that many classes practise this form. 'Ha', meaning sun, and 'tha', meaning moon, join to mean 'union', and the practice is designed to unite physical and spiritual harmony, and promote good physical health.

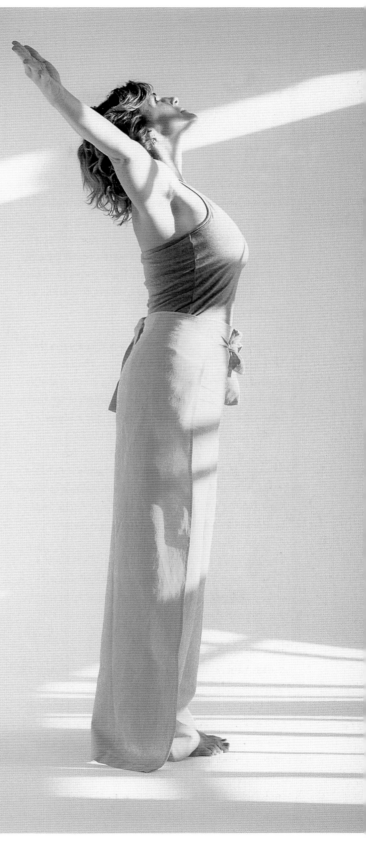

LEFT AND RIGHT **Yoga sequences, such as Sun Salutations, can help you to stretch and wind down for bed – and exercise performed throughout the day aids bedtime rest, too.**

- Iyengar yoga is very precise, with 12 tightly controlled postures. It can appear slow and seemingly straightforward to the untrained eye, but it takes time to master and to find the correct balance. It is excellent for muscle tone, posture and peace of mind.

- Kundalini yoga includes chanting and breath work as well as postures. It is said to be the best form for those looking for a spiritual element. It is also good for prenatal women and those after a youthful appearance.

- Sivananda and Jivamukti yoga are more meditative forms, and include an incense-scented ritual. Clearing the mind of stress is integral to these forms of yoga, so it is good for those hoping to alleviate worries and negative thought cycles.

- The most athletic form of yoga is Astanga yoga, which offers a cardiovascular workout. It has fat-burning and toning results, but is very demanding and not always ideal for a beginner. It is, however, excellent for those with experience and who are looking for a bigger challenge.

- Bikram yoga uses the principle that heat will help aid movement and flexibility. The room is heated to around 38°C (100°F), and you sweat out all your toxins while getting your body into some amazing positions.

Unwinding the body is essential if you want to get a good night's sleep, so the following basic yoga posture for relaxation should help free up your mind and body.

The Corpse

In yoga this pose is often practised between especially difficult poses and used to take the muscles and mind into a place of deep relaxation.

Lie on the floor with your legs slightly apart and your arms slightly outstretched. You should feel utterly natural, as if you have just flopped down on the grass in the sunshine. Avoid pointing your toes or clenching your fists. The back of your hands should be touching the floor and your palms should

point skyward. You may find that your muscles twitch or you want to stretch out your limbs, and this is the tension in your muscles making itself known. To combat this, try to imagine that you are extremely heavy and that the floor is supporting you. You can lie for as long as you like, but stay for at least five minutes. This is also a useful pose for meditation (see page 80).

INVITING PARTNERS TO THE SANCTUARY: ADVICE FOR LOVERS

Around two-thirds of us do not regularly sleep alone. Sometimes, however, our sleep problems mean we don't sleep together at all – in all senses of the word. Sleep problems are infectious; lying next to someone with sleep difficulties can mean that we soon end up sleepless, too.

One of the first areas to suffer when we are overtired is our sex life. Physical exhaustion and emotional hurt from unpleasant exchanges as a result of short fuses may leave us defensive and shaken. These upsets are just some of the reasons intimacy is neglected. The benefits of physical intimacy and an active sex life are well documented. Sex relieves stress and boosts our immune systems. By making it a rewarding part of our lives again, we can experience a renewal in our physical energy and our relationships.

Making Time

We are often so busy trying to make the most of our free time, because of demanding schedules, that time alone together becomes low on our list of priorities. Refusing a dinner invitation to stay in together alone, not always eating in front of the TV in a distracted daze after a long day, and asking the simple question, 'How was your day?', are all ways

RIGHT **Bed is a naturally intimate place that can also be used as a private retreat for couples where they can connect emotionally as well as physically.**

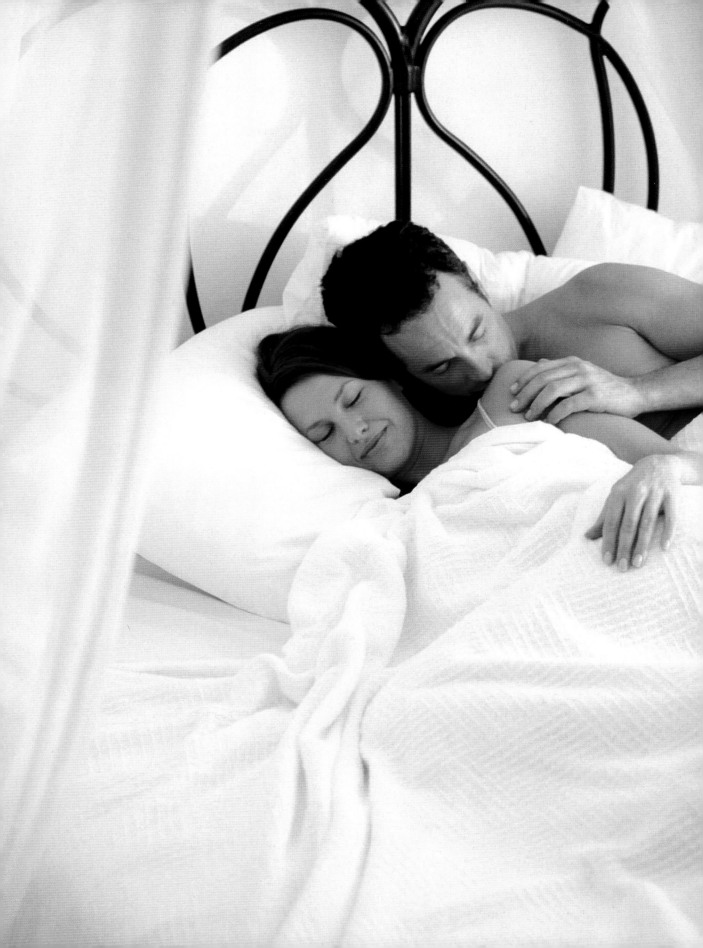

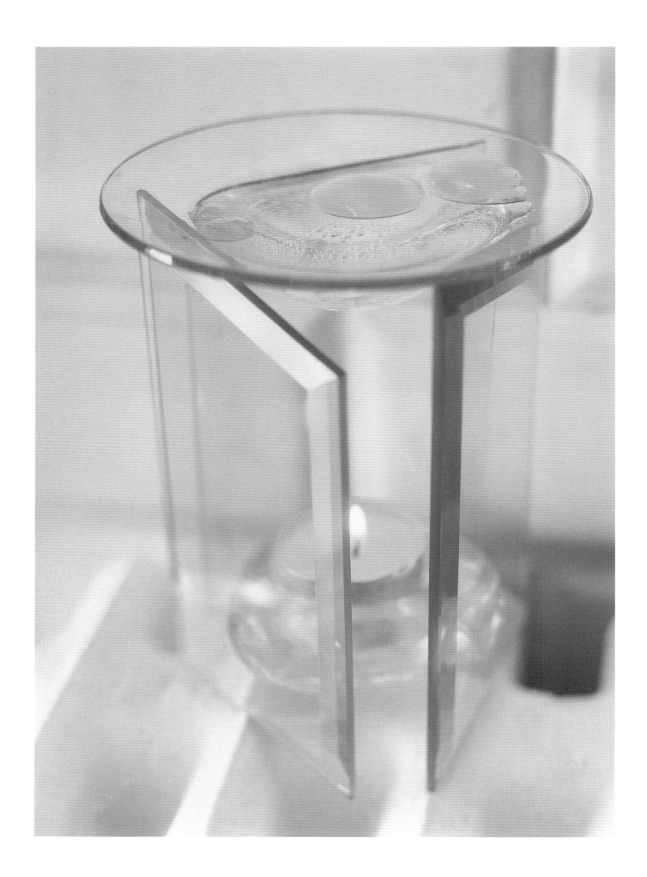

of getting your relationship back on track. Take advantage of our 24-hour society and get your groceries delivered so that you can spend Saturday morning in bed, instead of trailing round the supermarket. You have to put time and talking back at the top of your list in order to rediscover the desired level of intimacy.

Deploy the Aphrodisiacs

Assuming you have followed the earlier advice on making your bedroom a serene and sensuous space, you are now ready to use the rest of the tactics in the lover's campaign.

Before They Get Home

Take a relaxing bath with 3–5 drops of oils of lavender or mandarin oil in it before your lover gets home. Then put on something you know they like and that you feel good wearing. Essential rose mixed as body oil is said to heal matters of the heart and release anger at the self and others, including the feeling of betrayal or resentment. It replaces those negative feelings with ones of love and affection – great if you have been arguing.

On the Table

A dinner away from the clamour of a restaurant is a clear sign that you have something special in mind, and anticipation is wonderfully arousing. Try serving aphrodisiac foods, such as asparagus, oysters, celery or parsnips, ginger or cinnamon. Even if your loved one isn't sensitive to them, the message you send by serving them can be an aphrodisiac in itself.

LEFT **Burning oils is a subtle way of changing the mood. Your partner will also start to associate the scent with your romantic intentions.**

RIGHT **Use musky, heady scents, such as cedar, sandalwood and ylang ylang, to create a sensual and relaxed atmosphere in the bedroom.**

Seductive Scents

As smell is the most evocative of all the senses, aromatic oils, candles and incense can be very effective in initiating a mood for romance and intimacy. Jasmine, rose, patchouli, orange, sandalwood, rosewood and ylang ylang are an ideal accompaniment to seduction. Use oils in a burner or make up a massage blend for you both. Massage is a great way to make each other feel valued and central to each other's world and can be an effective prelude to lovemaking (see also pages 78–9). The more you use it, the more your mind will associate it with romance. Try this blend of essential oils to promote tenderness and connection:

2 drops of geranium
2 drops of cedarwood
3 drops of ylang ylang
3 drops of lavender
10 drops of a carrier oil of your choice, such as olive, sunflower or almond oil.

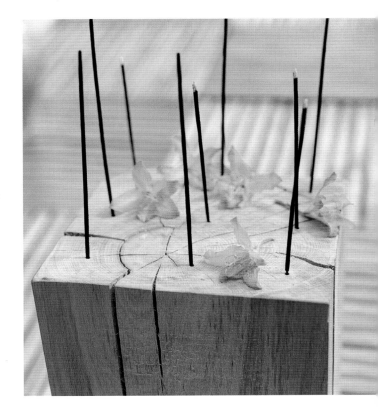

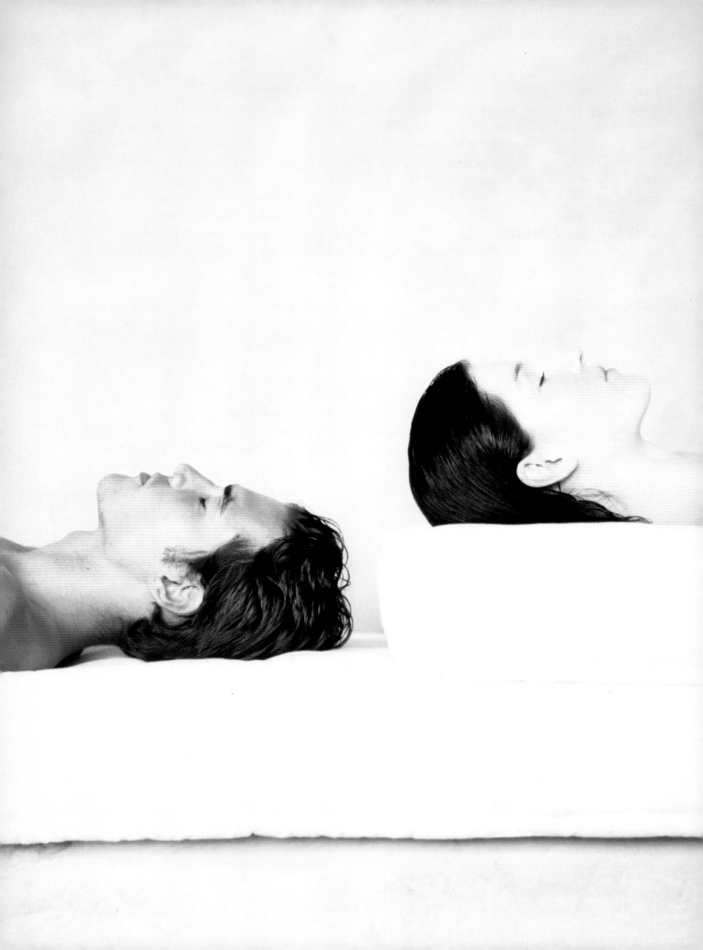

5 Holistic Therapies

FOR MANY PEOPLE, alternatives to traditional Western medical practice are becoming increasingly popular. Some of the positive aspects of using holistic therapies is that they are all natural and offer treatment without side effects or drug dependency.

Among the many alternative therapies you may find suitable in the fight against insomnia and other sleep-related disorders are aromatherapy, homeopathy, acupressure, acupuncture and Western medical herbalism.

When choosing any form of treatment, however, you must always make sure your practitioner is aware of any health-related factors, such as kidney or liver disease, pregnancy, Alzheimer's disease, or other medication you may be using to help with your condition, such as antidepressants. Natural, alternative treatments are not entirely innocuous and could affect, or be detrimentally affected by, any of these factors, or indeed by taking another homeopathic remedy. Make sure you find a registered professional to practise these treatments; details are listed on pages 156–7. And do be cautious of the many homeopathic remedies on the market advertised as natural – always buy from a well-respected source and follow the manufacturer's advice fully.

LEFT **Looking for new natural ways to improve your sleep will help you counteract the feelings of helpless that can accompany insomnia.**

SIMPLE ADVICE TO HELP YOU SLEEP

Before moving on to look at the various treatments that professionals can offer, here are a few simple, no-expense ways you can try to improve your sleep yourself.

- Make sure you go to bed and wake up at the same time every day. This helps programme the body and lets it prepare for the hour when you will want to retire.

- Switch on your answerphone and switch off your telephones at least 45 minutes before you go to bed. This will make sure you don't end up caught in a lengthy chat with a long-distance friend.

- Have a milky drink, herbal tea or sleepy snack before you go to bed, and practise other pre-sleep rituals (see pages 73–84).

- Don't toss and turn if you cannot sleep, as this can have a stimulating effect on the body and mind, working you up into even more of an agitated state. Try lying on your back and – working upwards from your feet – tense and release every muscle in your body while breathing deeply. Repeat this for as long as you need to.

- Zone your time and manage it. If you haven't finished a chore, set it aside and learn to move on to the next thing. Stress management is essential for good rest.

- Rather than lying there and getting frustrated, if you can't sleep, get up. Catch up with the ironing, do the washing up, anything as long as its boring – avoid re-stimulating your brain, however, by reading or watching TV.

- If random noises are disturbing you, put on a radio on low level to make soft monotonous noise that drowns the other noises out.

- Exercise is great for promoting sleep, but don't do it too close to bedtime as it will increase your metabolism and overstimulate your brain.

- If you still haven't slept well, resist the urge to sleep in longer than normal. Getting up on schedule keeps your body in its normal wake-up routine.

- Keep a sleep diary to stop you from obsessing. This will help you to spot whether there is a pattern emerging. For example, do you find yourself unable to sleep the night before important meetings or after working very late? Sleep diaries often show that although the diarist feels as if they have been awake all night, this is rarely true and the journal will help give you a more hopeful perspective.

- If you still have trouble falling asleep night after night, or constantly suffer from daytime tiredness, you might have a serious sleep disorder. At this point it is advisable to seek more advice from your doctor.

BELOW **A sleep diary is an excellent way of spotting potential causes of restlessness, such as drinking coffee or exercising too late in the day. It also enables you to write down your worries and release them from your mind.**

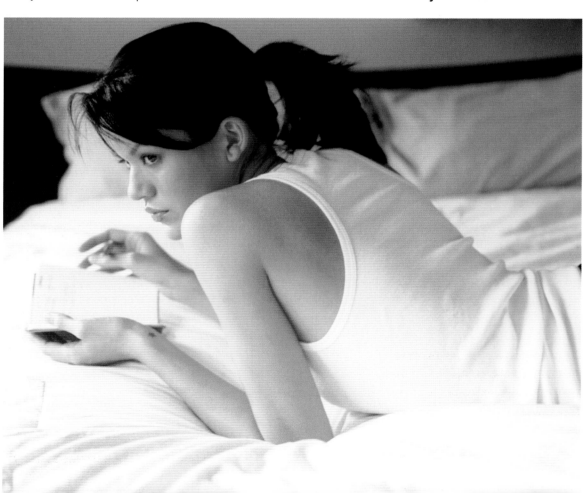

CONVENTIONAL CURES

For sleep problems, your GP may have offered a prescription sleeping drug. Most of the drugs will belong to a group known as benzodiazepines, which came into use in the 1960s and include the now-famous Valium. They can lower anxiety levels, a major cause of sleeplessness, by inhibiting the chemical action of the neurotransmitters. This slows the flow of information from one cell in the brain to another and quells the anxiety that speeds this process up. These drugs come in short-, medium- and long-acting forms and can have an effect from a few hours to a few days. All of them reduce the amount of time it takes to fall asleep and can reduce the number of night-time wakings. Unfortunately, they lose their potency with continued use so doses must be increased, and they are highly addictive. Side effects can include dependency (with withdrawal symptoms), impaired reactions and nightmares.

There is a new generation of drugs that were introduced in the 1990s, the most common of which are Zaleplon and Zolpidem, which are much safer to use. These speed the onset of sleep, but have a short life of up to four hours. Headaches and drowsiness can still occur as side effects.

ACUPUNCTURE AND ACUPRESSURE

Acupuncture has evolved over thousands of years. Like all forms of Chinese healing traditions, it is based on the concept of maintaining balance and harmony within the body. Studies have reported that it is helpful for insomnia, showing that those who have received it fell asleep faster and slept more soundly. It can also relieve insomnia by addressing other issues, such as illness or anxiety that can disturb sleep patterns.

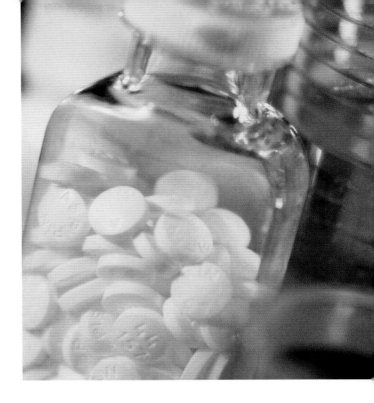

ABOVE **Advances in traditional drug therapy offer safer alternatives to early sleeping pills, which were addictive, increased tolerance and left users with a hungover feeling the next morning.**

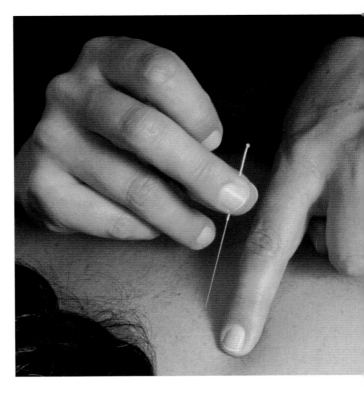

RIGHT **Acupuncture approaches the body as a whole, treating the possible causes of insomnia as well as relieving the symptoms.**

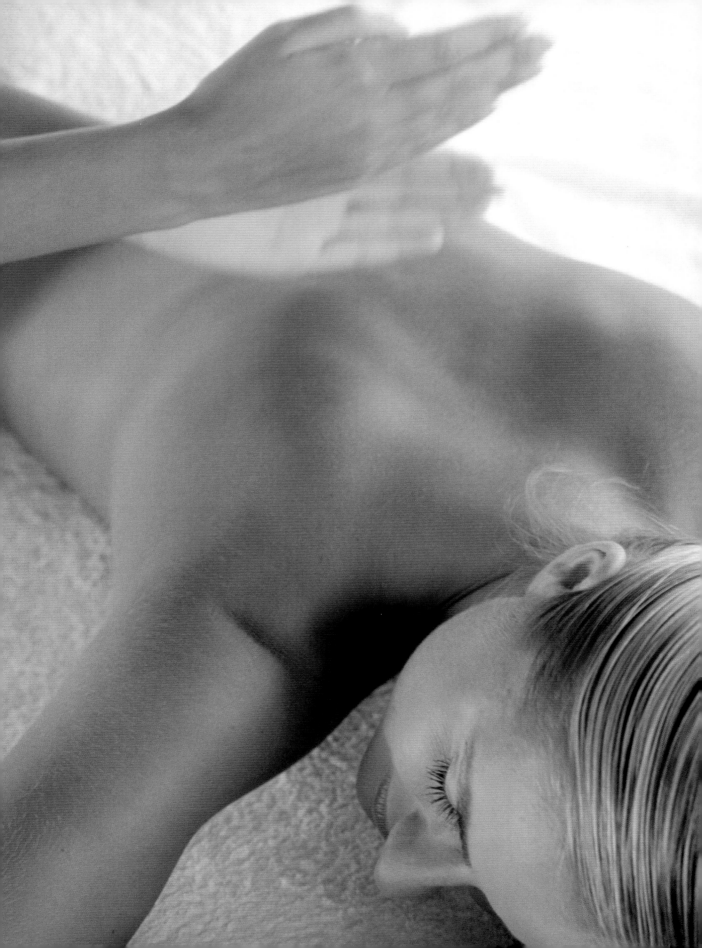

Acupuncture works on the principle that illness and disease are a result of the disruption, or blockage of the flow of chi or qi (life energy). Qi consists of equal and opposite qualities – yin and yang – and when these become unbalanced illness may result. By inserting fine needles into the channels of energy, an acupuncturist can stimulate the body's own healing response. The flow of qi can be disturbed by a number of factors. These include emotional states such as anxiety, stress, anger, fear or grief, poor nutrition, weather conditions, poisons, infections, hereditary factors and trauma. To release the flow, needles are inserted into points along the meridians (energetic pathways) of the body. There are more than 350 points on the meridians of the body, so the acupuncturist will determine which to use by questioning and examining the patient. This method ensures that the cause of the sleeplessness, and not just the effect, is treated.

Acupressure works on the same principles, but is noninvasive. It works to relieve, calm and enliven the body and mind and its most frequently found form is shiatsu massage. Zero-balancing is a newer addition to the acupressure arts, but this also encourages harmony within the body. Reflexology works on a similar principle and dates back to ancient Egypt, India and China. It concentrates on massaging specific points of the feet, which correspond to organs and systems in the body, thus encouraging the body to rebalance – it can be particularly soothing for those with sleep difficulties. Each therapy tends to last about an hour, and you should talk through the resulting sensations; for example, some patients may feel weepy, tired or faintly nauseous after reflexology or energy work, but this a perfectly natural indicator that the treatment is working and changes are occurring.

LEFT **The powerful techniques involved in massage and shiatsu – a form of acupressure – can create a profound feeling of restfulness and calm, reducing the tension in the muscles and the mind.**

AROMATHERAPY

We all use aromatherapy, in its most basic form, every day. The smell of baking bread, a rosewater perfume or an aversion to bad smells are all powerful stimulators of memory and sense. In its technical application, it is an effective and soothing way to balance moods and manage energy and it is an effective way to relieve sleeplessness. The oils provoke a variety of different responses by stimulating the olfactory organs, which are linked to the areas of the brain that control emotions, causing a series of chemical reactions effecting a physical or emotional change in the body. If you don't appreciate a particular scent, it won't relax you and you should try something else. Oils can be used by adding them to a bath, burning them in a diffuser or using them in a compress. For sleep problems, they can be particularly effective in the form of massage, especially if your poor sleep is due to muscle tension.

BELOW **An oil burner or candle can fill a room with an ambient fragrance that can help promote a restful night's sleep.**

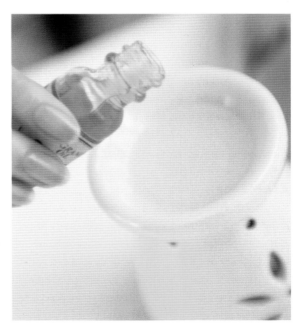

Always buy pure oils, rather than synthetic oils. Most essential oils require a 'carrier' oil, such as olive, sunflower or almond oil, and should be mixed before use in massage as they are highly concentrated and can cause skin irritation. Their potency means you only need a very small amount. For massage on adults, 28 ml (1 fl oz) of carrier oil should have only 12–15 drops of essential oil added. When using it in the bath, 10–12 drops of essential oil should be used. The water temperature should be sufficiently hot to ensure that the oil mixes fully with the water. This has the dual effect of helping the oil to soak into the skin and producing an oil-enhanced steam that is breathed in – make sure the doors and windows are closed to encourage maximum inhalation. When properly stored in a cool, dark place, essential oils can last for years. Once they are combined with a carrier oil, however, they will turn rancid within three months, so use them up.

The following essential oils are known to be effective for aiding a good night's rest. In their dried form some can also be used to stuff 'sleep pillows', which will promote rest as you sleep. Herbs such as basil and marjoram can be ingested in food dishes or made into teas.

BASIL

This herb can promote calm and rest for those suffering from nervous insomnia or fatigue. It is also regarded as an aphrodisiac, which is ideal if you are feeling too tired to even contemplate sex. The flower heads and leaves can be used in cooking, so ingest their benefits with a refreshing mozzarella, tomato and basil salad.

CLARY SAGE

This is regarded as an all-round panacea, and supports the central nervous system in many of its duties. From fatigue, depression and headaches, it can relieve many of the problems associated with poor sleep. Its benefits can be gained from eating it fresh, as well as in an essential oil form. Add it to salads, or stuff chicken breast with it.

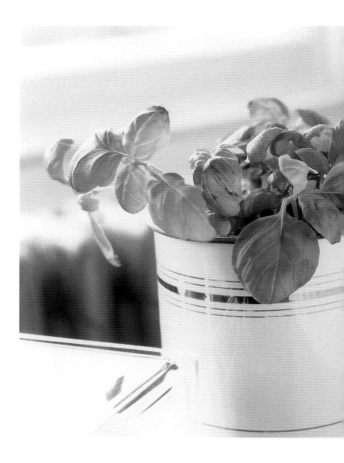

ABOVE **Basil will grow happily on a window sill, providing you with a fresh supply always at hand to use in a salad.**

FRANKINCENSE

This is an ancient and widely used gum resin from Africa and the Middle East that can aid meditation. Place a few drops on a piece of cotton wool or in a small dish of water near a warm radiator before you start to meditate. Inhale the fragrance deeply throughout your session.

GERANIUM

Use geranium essential oil for renewing and reviving a tired mind. It is also a great antiseptic and insect repellent and one of the most useful and important aromatherapy oils. Use it in self-massage to fight the fatigue caused by poor sleep or stressful demands.

The powerful effects of essential oils can
be used to make massage and bath oils
that ease away any stresses and strains.

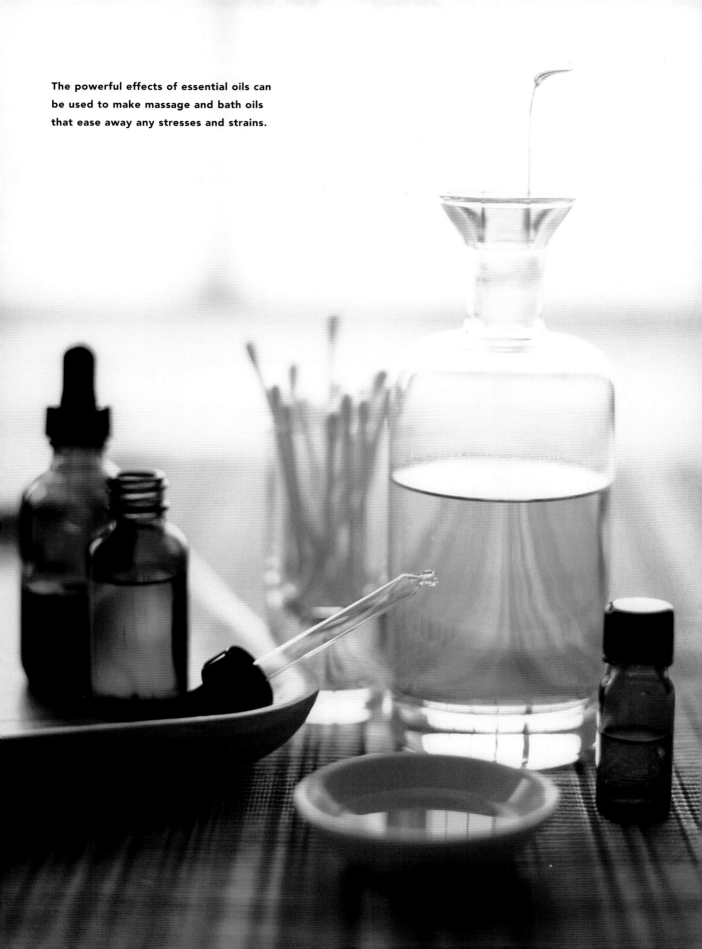

LAVENDER

Amazingly effective in encouraging sleep and relaxation. In studies published in the medical journal, *The Lancet*, lavender has been shown to be as effective as sleeping pills for the elderly. A great way to promote rest is to add a few drops to your linen spray when you are ironing your sheets. This way you can subtly infuse your whole sleep space with the scent. You can always freshen up the scent by spraying directly onto your pillow. Alternatively, put a few sprigs in the linen cupboard. Lavender has traditionally been used to provide relaxation and drowsiness, but be careful, using more than 1–2 drops can have the opposite effect.

MELISSA OR LEMON BALM

This has a sedative effect when the fragrance is inhaled. Originally from Southern Europe, it was spread by the Romans and it is ideal for insomnia, and sleep enemies such as depression, migraines and PMS. It is also very effective as a tea or in foods – the lemony flavour is great for soups and desserts.

MANDARIN

A member of the orange family, the oil comes from the skin of the fruit rather than the flowers. The bromine content, which calms the nervous system, is very high, so following dinner with a couple of these for dessert will have a sedative effect on anxious people. It can also be used in the bath.

MARJORAM

This has a powerful sedative effect and is great if you are sleeping badly owing to nervous tension or are just generally tired. It can be used in a massage oil or oil burner, mixed with a drop of orange oil on a tissue by the bed or as a soothing drink in its dried form – a pinch of marjoram and one of dried

RIGHT Some ceramic burners are used with scented tealights instead of oils, but don't forget to extinquish the flame before you sleep.

lime flowers in hot water, half an hour before going to bed, will encourage sleep.

NEROLI

Originating from the flower of the orange tree, neroli oil can be used to treat depression, anxiety and insomnia, either in a relaxing bath, as a drink or just in its fruit form. Using it in hot water and steaming the skin can treat acne and poor skin conditions, which may often be exacerbated by poor sleep.

PETITGRAIN

Another product from the orange tree, this is derived from the leaves, twigs and unripe fruit. It is a very effective relaxant and has similar effects to neroli. It is especially good if you are coming off tranquillizers, which may have been prescribed to treat insomnia symptoms. Like neroli, its benefits can also be gleaned from placing an orange plant in your room.

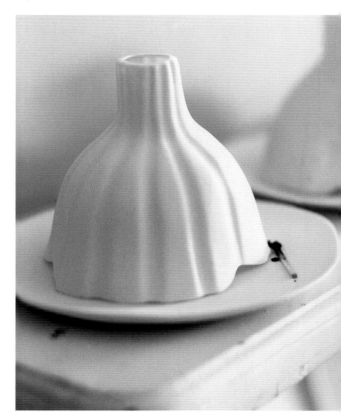

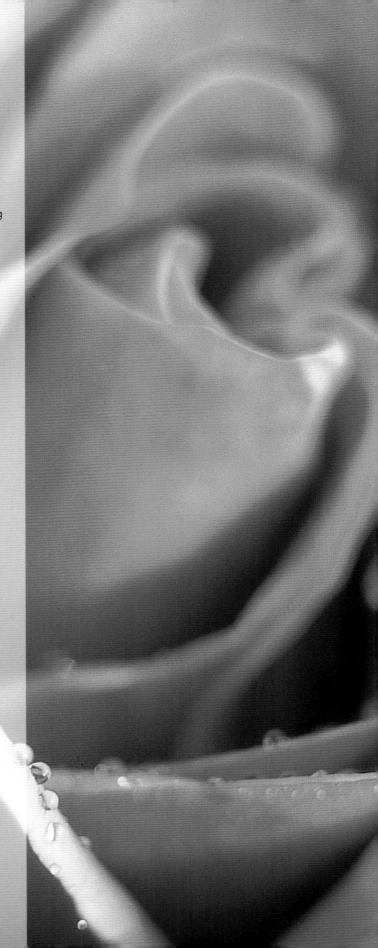

ROSE

This is particularly helpful for treating women who are suffering from insomnia due to anxiety or a nervous disposition. Whether massaging rose oil into the solar plexus, drinking a rose infusion tea or putting it in the bath, it is an easy oil to work into your routine as it has such a pretty scent. It can be used to fragrance desserts or as a salad dressing when mixed with white wine vinegar.

SANDALWOOD

This has been used in Ayurvedic, Asian and Arab forms of treatment for centuries, and is very calming. Keeping sheets in a sandalwood chest can have a very relaxing effect when you put them on the bed. It is also a good aid for meditation.

TANGERINE

The fruity, sweet scent is calming and ideal for treating not only anxiety and insomnia but also muscle pain and ageing skin.

Insomnia Blend

Blend these oils for a truly restful sleep:

  10 drops of roman camomile
  5 drops of clary sage
  5 drops of bergamot.

  Blend the oils well in a clean, dark-coloured glass bottle. Add one to two drops to a tissue and place it inside your pillow to aid you in falling asleep. If you prefer to make a diffuser blend that you can enjoy during the hour before bedtime, make a blend with a ratio of two drops of Roman camomile to one drop of clary sage to one drop of bergamot and add to your diffuser.

RIGHT **Essential rose oil is especially effective for women seeking relief from anxiety. Wonderfully versatile, it can be used in tea, massage oil or even cooking.**

HOMEOPATHY

Used by an estimated thirty million people in Europe, homeopathy is designed to work with your body through a holistic system of healing, which works on physical and emotional symptoms. A homeopath will ask you about your lifestyle, worries and hopes as well as your physical symptoms. To stimulate your body's own healing process, a remedy that is tailored especially for you is prescribed. The healing begins from within your body, strengthening your health and immune system without the danger of damaging side effects. No synthetic products are used, but you should avoid eating, drinking, smoking or using toothpaste for 20 minutes after taking a homeopathic medicine.

Conventional and homeopathic medicine can be taken at the same time, but if you are unsure always consult your healthcare provider. The following treatments are most useful for sleep-related problems.

COCCULUS

Ideal for insomnia following a tiring long journey or being in a hectic, smoky atmosphere. It is also recommended for anxiety and sleep that is disturbed by nightmares.

ACID PHOSPHORUS

Helps to overcome mental and physical debility caused by a prolonged bout of grief, whatever the cause.

IGNATIA

This can help those who have received shocking news that consequently leads to disturbed sleep. Rapid mood swings, weepiness or tiredness can also be alleviated.

CAMOMILLA

Useful for sleeplessness in crying, angry and restless children, especially when they are teething or suffering from colic. Sometimes the child may demand things, then refuse them, and is hot, thirsty or irritable.

COFFEA

For physical restlessness and insomnia when the mind is churning up difficult thoughts and worries from the day. The alertness of the mind can result in light and interrupted unrefreshing sleep; coffea will slow down a racing mind.

KALI. PHOSPHORUS

Can be used to treat weakness and tiredness, especially after worry, excitement or overwork.

NUX VOMICA

When the mind is overstimulated or strained, this can help calm your thoughts – anger at being unable to sleep is often one of the symptoms. It can aid in regularizing sleep and it also helps sleep patterns that are disturbed by too many stimulants, such as alcohol, coffee and stress.

LACHESIS

Repetitive insomnia can result in a fear of going to bed, which this treatment can ease. If you suffer from menstruation-related insomnia or jolting limbs when trying to fall asleep, this remedy helps both complaints.

ARSENICUM ALBUM

Use this to tackle the unpleasant experience of waking in the middle of the night fretting over problems. This sign of anxiety responds well to this treatment.

ARNICA

Can aid the exhaustion that follows extended physical and mental effort, and can also help with jet lag if taken before the journey.

RIGHT **Homeopathic treatments can be used on their own, or in unison, to help treat very specific types of insomnia and its causes, aiding in improving the quality of sleep. Ask a practitioner for advice on prescribing and combining the remedies.**

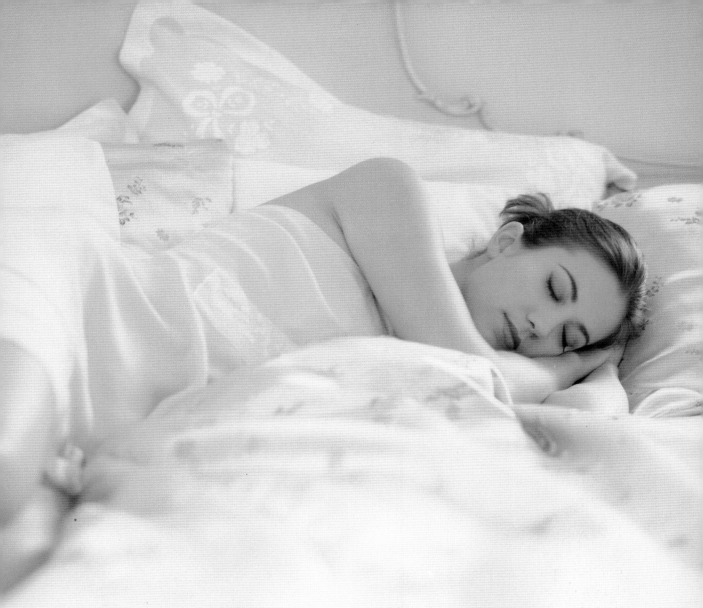

WESTERN HERBAL MEDICINE

Herbalism has its roots in the indigenous practices of the British Isles, Europe and North America. A significant proportion of orthodox Western medicines were originally derived from herbal medicines, but Western herbal medicine also has a holistic attitude to health. The patient, rather than the disease or condition, is the focus here. The background to the patient's condition is assessed through family and health history and lifestyle, and therapy is directed at the causes, not just the presenting symptoms. The practitioner then uses this information to assess the vitality and constitution of the patient, using this for the choice of herbs in the prescription. Prescriptions may vary substantially between individual patients with apparently similar conditions, and the herbal treatment is used as part of a bigger approach to understanding effects such as lifestyle and nutrition.

There are a huge number of conventional over-the-counter sleep medications. These have their side effects and price to pay, not least of which is dependency. One of the key advantages of herbal medicines is that they are not believed to interfere with the sleep stages, something that can occur with conventional, chemical ones. Various plants are said to have sedative effects, such as hops, skullcap and black cohosh, and the effectiveness of these

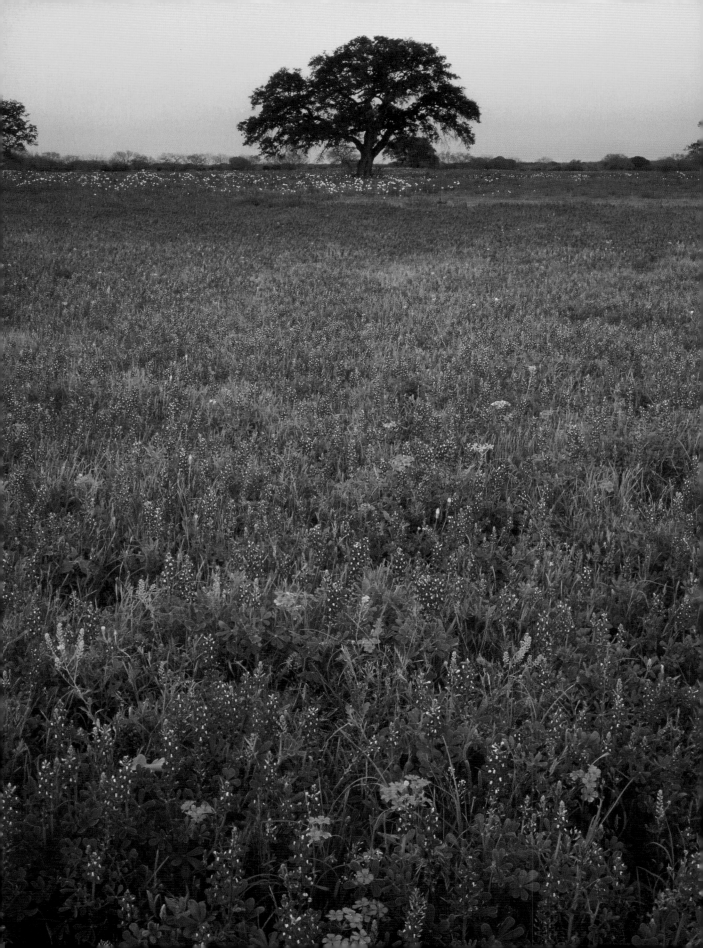

plants is very much down to the individual – a degree of experimentation can bring about the right blend for you, but most herbal supplements carry a mix of them, usually in conjunction with the most effective, which is valerian. A well-known hypnotic and sedative, it comes from the root of the heliotrope (*Valerian officinalis*) plant. It appears to improve sleep gradually, although it is also effective when taken for occasional insomnia. It is one of the most potent natural treatments available and can be taken alone, although many over-the-counter preparations mix it with a combination of other sedatives such as hops, passionflower and lemon balm. A good example of this is the tincture *avena sativa* compound, an effective sleep medicine comprising a number of the herbs, including passionflower, valerian and hops. It should be taken in water just before going to bed.

BACH FLOWER ESSENCES

Flower remedies were originally the brainchild of Dr Edward Bach, who studied medicine at the University College Hospital, London. In the 1930s, after developing an interest in alternative health, he gave up his lucrative Harley Street practice and left London, deciding to devote the rest of his life to a new system of medicine that he believed could be sourced from nature.

Bach found that when he treated the feelings and personalities of his patients, their unhappiness and physical distress was alleviated. This 'unlocked' the natural healing potential already in their bodies, allowing them to recover. His system is composed of 38 tinctures. Each is aimed at a particular mental state or emotion and all have a specific 'vibration', which can be used alone or together to treat different states of mind from panic to forgetfulness.

LEFT AND RIGHT **The natural world is our greatest resource for curing our illnesses and ailments, contributing to herbal medicines, flower remedies and beauty and spa salves and treatments.**

The emotions described are often quite specific; listed below are three recommendations for dealing with insomnia.

WHITE CHESTNUT
When your mind is so cluttered with thoughts that you are unable to fall asleep.

IMPATIENS
When you get irritated and impatient with yourself as you start counting the hours until the alarm clock goes off.

VERVAIN
When your mind is too wound up with plans and excitement to sleep.

If you are unsure which remedies are best for you, an alternative health practitioner can help you decide. You can then combine them in a single bottle, or use them individually and as you need. Each bottle has a pipette (dropper) to allow you to administer them exactly. They can also be added to water or the bath – you need to soak for 30 minutes if this is your preferred method.

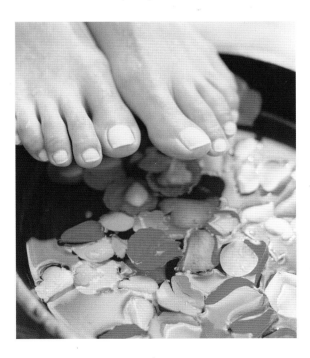

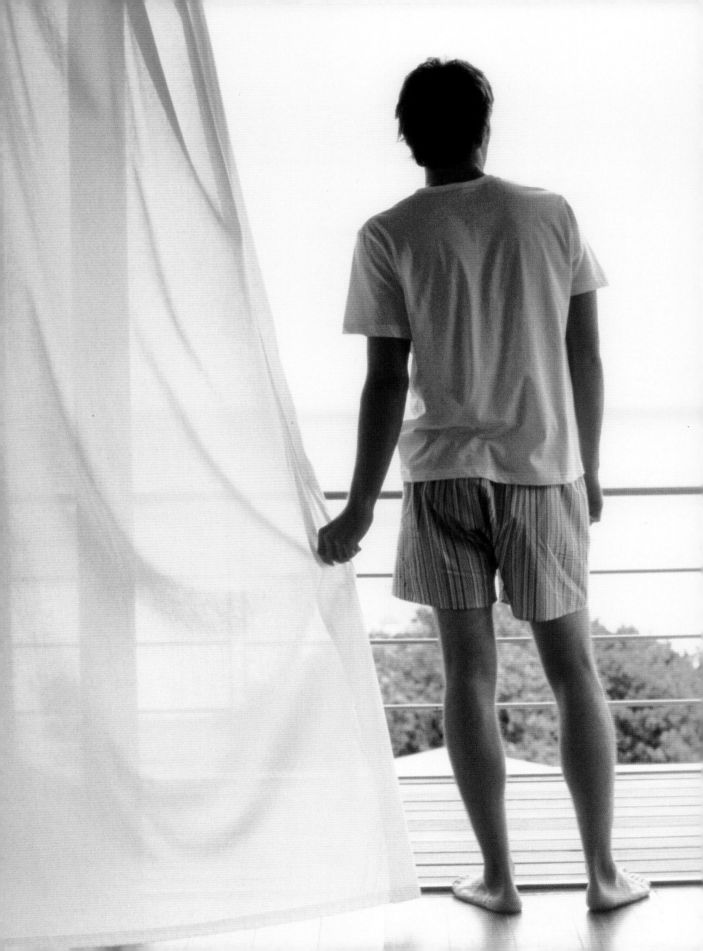

6 Fast-Track Strategies

SLEEP CAN BE WONDERFULLY restorative and renewing. A lack of it, however, can consume life with a range of deprivation symptoms. This section is designed to give you a practical helping hand for dealing with some of the most distressing and common complaints associated with poor sleep. If you are on medication or feel unsure about the suitability of a particular remedy, talk to your doctor, pharmacist or local alternative health practitioner about finding a combination that works. And keep experimenting; we're all different and have changing needs, so we can always benefit from trying out new remedies.

ANXIETY

At one end of the scale, anxiety can feel mildly troubling and slightly disconcerting; at the other end it can be totally incapacitating and isolating. Anxiety can become an ever-present problem; you feel unable to handle the feelings of panic and unease and it often seems to have no rational trigger. It can be the result of one singularly traumatic event, such as the death of a relative, redundancy or end of a relationship, or it can be a more gradual process, such as a continually stressful work environment. Free-floating anxiety is a continual undercurrent that is not attributable to any specific situation or reasonable danger, and can be associated with panic and panic attacks.

LEFT **Understanding the symptoms that enable you to recognize a particular condition can help you select the most effective form of treatment to alleviate the problem.**

Ideally, the most effective approach to the management of anxiety would be the removal of the source of stress, a rebalancing therapy and support from a good diet and a willing ear. In reality, this isn't always possible, but the following methods of treatment can offer relief. If you are concerned at any time, do approach a heath practitioner to ensure you find the best solution. The conventional medical approach might offer some form of tranquillizer to break the cycle, but the problem with this can be a dependency. There are also many alternative treatments to consider.

Common Symptoms
- Palpitations
- Nausea
- Perspiration
- Digestive problems (diarrhoea or constipation)
- Light-headedness
- Tingling in the hands and arms
- Rapid shallow breathing
- Muscle discomfort

Breathing

Learning to master your breathing can be a great way to control feelings of anxiety and distress. When we feel panicked, we often take shallow, quick breaths. This leads to an imbalance between the carbon dioxide and oxygen in the bloodstream and makes the anxiety much worse. Diaphragmatic breathing, used in yoga, lets us pull air deep into our lower lungs to address the imbalance of oxygen and carbon dioxide in our bodies and calm us down. See page 82 for how to master this technique.

Reset Your Mind

'Reframing', taking the same set of facts and applying a different meaning to them, is a technique often employed by psychotherapists to help clients get a more positive perspective.

For example, if you have an argument with a friend, rather than blame yourself for it, try to see it as a chance to change the dynamics of how you relate to each other. In its most basic form, it is about looking for the positive in everything. Most people can improve their perspectives by reprogramming their minds to think of themselves as fortunate. Start by resisting the temptation to relive your past failures and worries. It can dampen your spirit and

BELOW **The feelings of frustration and helplessness that accompany the sensation of lying awake counting the passing hours can be relieved by learning simple deep-breathing and relaxation techniques.**

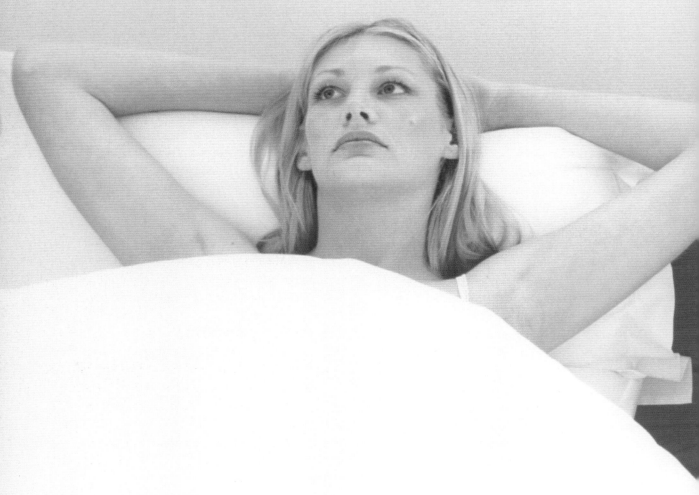

encourage you to stress over difficulties during your day. Get things in perspective, look for opportunities in disaster and see taking chances as a natural part of the process of fulfilling your dreams – this will help you to persist in the face of failure. The more often you do it, the quicker it becomes your default mechanism.

Aromatherapy

It's important, when you are suffering from anxiety or stress, to make sure you have a safe space in which you can unwind. Make time every night to have a soothing bath, at least an hour before you go to bed as this will help you sleep. Add a few drops of essential camomile, melissa or jasmine oil to the water to treat the lack of confidence that can result from anxiety.

Diet

Stimulants, such as tea, coffee and sugar-laden products, may seem comforting but they will only exaggerate your feelings of angst. Tryptophan is ideal in this situation, so look for genuine comfort foods that contain it (see pages 51–2). Bananas are a great snack, as is a turkey and lettuce sandwich or a handful of almonds. Replace regular tea with caffeine-free roibosh or soothing camomile. And don't leave long gaps between meals; you may feel too anxious to eat but you will only make your symptoms worse by making your sugar levels unstable. If camomile tea isn't for you, try an alternative such as lime flower (also known as linden), passionflower or valerian. A little honey can be a nice addition, but not too much as it is a sugar and should be used in moderation to keep your blood sugar levels stable.

Essential Supplements

Vitamin B complex is good for overall health and helps the body cope with the stress you may be under. Kava kava is a natural sedative and relaxant, and as such a good alternative to tranquillizers (never take both kava kava and tranquillizers together).

Homeopathy

ACID PHOSPHORUS

Free-floating anxiety can be debilitating, and this treatment can help very sensitive people who need a lot of reassurance.

ACONITE

Good for anxiety that has been caused by unsettling news or a distressing event. Symptoms of mental and physical restlessness and panic attacks respond well to this treatment.

GELSEMIUM

Anxiety that has developed gradually over time should be treated with this remedy. People who suffer from long-term anxiety may become withdrawn and irritable and suffer headaches as side effects – gelsemium should address all these needs.

ARSENICUM ALBUM

A worried or tense expression often signifies the need for this remedy, which treats patients who are pressurizing themselves over achieving goals and perfectionism. Sleeplessness, irritability, restlessness and sensitivity to the cold can also accompany this obsessive anxiety.

CALC CARB SP

This helps those who are mentally, physically and emotionally exhausted from overwork and stress, who can become anxious, apprehensive and occasionally confused, all factors that lead to disturbed sleep and being run down.

Flower Remedies

Keep a bottle of Bach Rescue Remedy with you at all times to cope with the symptoms of anxiety. As soon as you begin to feel unsettled or experience the signs of panic and fear, take a few drops in a glass of water or straight under your tongue. Other remedies that might help are white chestnut, for calm and clarity of mind, and rock rose, which helps to allay feelings of fear.

LACK OF CONCENTRATION, FOCUS AND MOTIVATION

An inability to concentrate or focus and a general feeling of disinterest are common in those suffering from poor sleep. These symptoms are often compounded by the sufferer's lack of concern about the outcome of their poor performance as they are simply too tired to care. This can cause serious problems in situations where close attention is demanded, such as driving or health and safety issues in the workplace.

The most effective way to improve this situation is to take a nap. Even 20 minutes is shown to improve concentration and make you more alert and capable of performing the tasks in hand.

Common Symptoms
- Dulled mental skills
- Forgetfulness
- Repetition of ineffective approaches
- Inflexibility
- Bad decision-making
- Impetuous decisions

Diet
Avoid self-medicating with too much caffeine and sugar, which just gives you quick highs of energy followed by troughs of exhaustion. A little dose of caffeine can focus your mind and give you a boost, but limit yourself to no more than three cups of tea a day, two of coffee. (Even though tea contains as much caffeine, it tends not to be served in such concentrated measures). Do not drink them after 5 pm or they will affect your ability to fall asleep and exacerbate the problem. Dehydration is a classic cause of bad concentration, so make sure you are getting enough water. Increase your intake to at least 2.5 litres (4¼ pints) a day. Start the day with porridge, a slow-release energy source that will help you focus. Eat lean meat and vegetables that are low in carbohydrates, such as green leafy vegetables, for lunch. This will help you through the afternoon dip in energy caused by the natural cycle of your circadian rhythm.

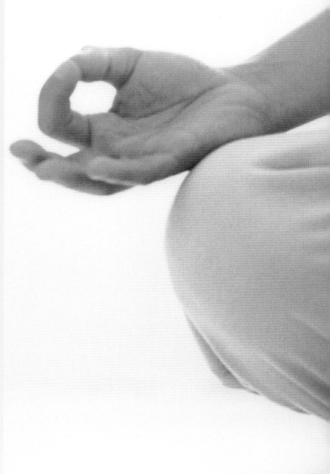

ABOVE **Inability to concentrate or care about the outcome of neglected projects is a classic sign of exhaustion, and can be helped immediately by a period of meditation or a short nap.**

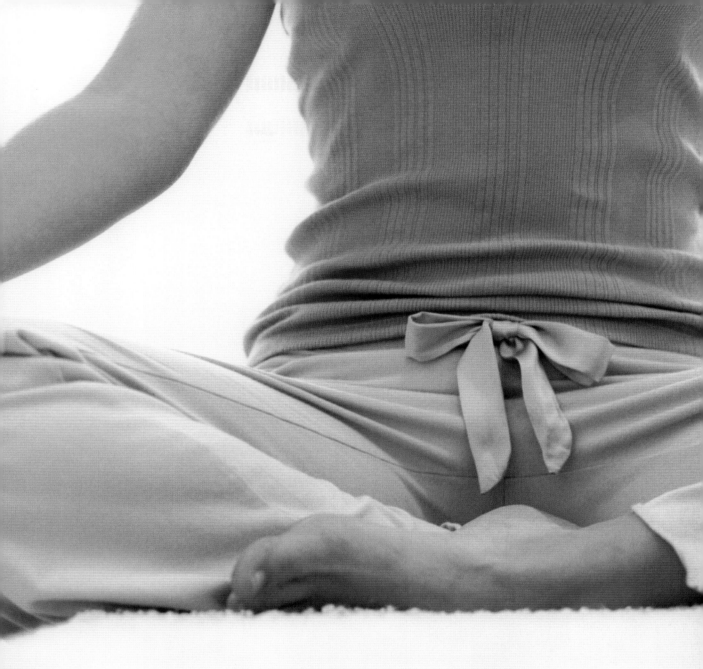

Aromatherapy

If you have a project you simply must finish or an important deadline, diffusing geranium oil in the room when you have to keep working late should help renew and refocus you.

Flower Remedies

Try the Bach Flower remedy white chestnut to regain clarity of mind and bring you back to the matters in hand.

Meditation

Simple exercises can focus your mind and clear distracted thoughts. See breathing, meditation and visualization on pages 80–2 for how to master these useful techniques.

Homeopathy

Arnica is helpful if taken before a long, tiring journey. It helps counter fatigue when you need to concentrate.

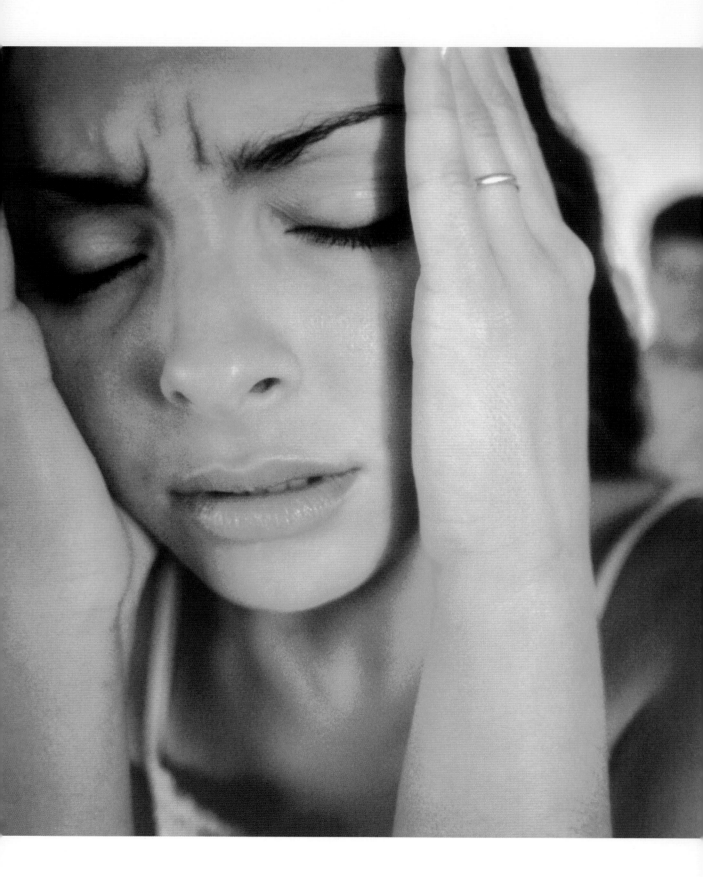

MOOD SWINGS

Anyone who has lived with a sleep-deprived person can attest to the presence of mood swings. As well as the physical feeling of being overtired, hormonal imbalances, which are exacerbated by lack of sleep, can also cause mood swings. This is often an integral part of other conditions, such as menopause and premenstrual syndrome/tension (PMS/PMT) in women. Hormone replacement therapy is usually offered for menopause and taking the contraceptive pill is sometimes recommended by doctors in order to regulate and alleviate symptoms of PMS.

Very tired people are also often found hanging around the coffee maker at the office, offering to buy snacks or looking exhausted just after lunch. This is because tiredness can induce cravings for a sugar hit, and one stimulant often quickly needs to be followed by another.

Common Symptoms

- Irritability
- Aggression
- Anger
- Sadness
- Exhaustion
- Feeling weepy and unable to cope
- Hot flushes
- Aches and pains
- Cravings
- Tendency to eat sweet, processed or snack foods; reliance on stimulants
- Energy slumps during the day

Aromatherapy

A feeling of being unappreciated can often come with mood swings, so making time for yourself is essential. Taking a hot bath with an aromatherapy candle is wonderfully indulgent. Also try adding a few drops of essential oil to the warm water to complement the candle, such as lavender, camomile, marjoram and/or frankincense.

Diet

High-fibre foods can help lessen mood swings caused by hormonal imbalance. Increase your water intake to 2.5 litres (4¼ pints) a day to help the fibre perform its duties properly. Eat chromium-rich foods, such as cheese, shellfish, baked beans and wholemeal bread, to help overcome the symptoms of hypoglycaemia (low blood sugar). Fresh fruit is a slow-releasing food that will stop you reaching for quick-fix, sugar-rich snacks.

Flower Remedies

The Bach Flower remedy white chestnut will help soothe and restore your clarity of mind when you are feeling unbalanced.

Supplement

Phytonutrient herbs, such as liquorice, that boost levels of oestrogen, and ginseng that helps balance the body's adrenal hormones (related to stress) can be used to balance hormone levels. Women who eat phytoestrogens, such as wheat, green and yellow vegetables, citrus fruits, oats and rhubarb, have fewer problems at menopause.

LEFT **Mood swings caused by lack of sleep are inevitable, yet incredibly hard to control, taxing relationships in every area of your life from work to romance.**

DAYTIME SLEEPINESS

Most people experience this to some degree as our natural circadian rhythm has a dip early afternoon. Everyone will have their own particular 'low' point, but it should pass by about 5 pm and be followed by a more energetic period in the evening. If you find yourself fighting sleep at your desk or nodding off in the supermarket, this is usually a sign that you are sleep-deprived. More serious sleep problems, like narcolepsy (see page 31) and sleep apnoea (see page 28) may be possible reasons, so if you are seriously concerned and altering your sleep routine and the number of hours you sleep is not resulting in an improvement, see your doctor. To check if your daytime sleepiness is a result of being sleep-deprived, check your Sleep Latency Period (see page 18).

In the battle against sleepiness, falling asleep could help. If you can barely keep your eyes open during the day, set aside a little time for a rejuvenating power nap. Even 20 minutes can help improve your performance and mood. Make sure it is no more than 20 minutes, though, or it will affect your night-time sleep. Even losing an hour a night over several nights will leave you with a sleep deficit that can result in daytime sleepiness, so prioritize your sleep until you have caught up.

Common Symptoms

- Lack of concentration
- Irritability
- An overwhelming desire to sleep
- Falling asleep less than 10 minutes after retiring to bed

Diet

Avoid refined carbohydrates, such as white bread, for lunch as it will emphasize the natural lull in your circadian rhythm. Opt for slow-releasing energy foods, such as porridge, for breakfast. Caffeine can give a boost, but avoid it after 5 pm as it will keep the cycle going.

BELOW **Mild daytime sleepiness is a natural effect of our inbuilt circadian rhythm, but an overwhelming desire suggests night-time sleep is poor quality.**

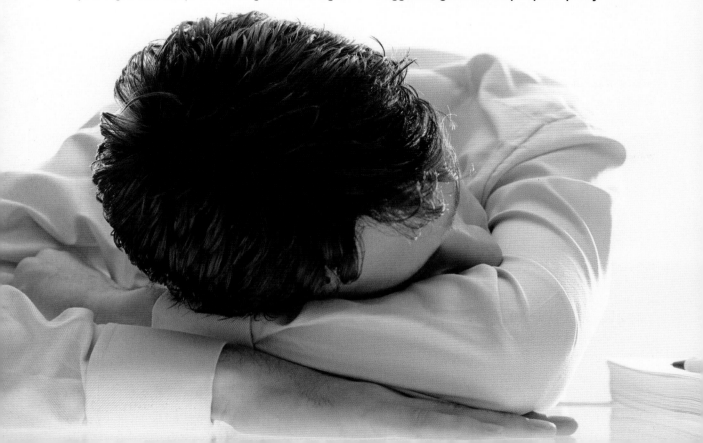

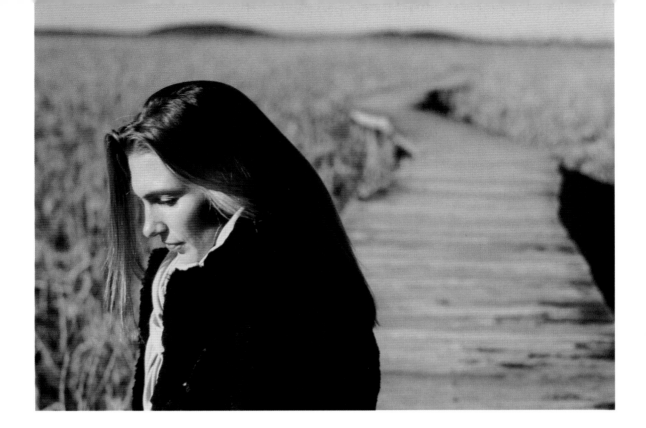

ABOVE **Depression is an isolating and distressing illness, but most cases can be radically alleviated with therapies, whether they are medical, alternative or counselling.**

DEPRESSION

Emotional resilience can be seriously impaired by lack of sleep, making you susceptible to depression. Whether the depression has been triggered by sleeplessness or the insomnia is a symptom of depression, the depression will be unlikely to lift without some intervention. If you are prescribed anti-depressants (usually an SSRI or serotonin reuptake inhibitor, the most famous being Prozac) you must ensure that any other treatments can be used safely with them, as they are not always compatible. An essential part of emerging from depression is talking. No matter whether or not you feel you want to discuss the origin of your depression, it can help to talk about the feeling of being depressed in itself. Talking can also alleviate symptoms of isolation, speed recovery and help resolve the issues that may have caused the depression in the first place.

Common Symptoms

- Disturbed sleep (such as insomnia or oversleeping)
- Anxiety
- Loss of appetite
- Poor concentration
- Loss of motivation
- Mood swings
- Lowered libido
- Negative thought cycles
- Hyperventilation

Aromatherapy

Essential oils, such as basil, marjoram, lemon balm, neroli, thyme and verbena are all known for their ability to help treat the symptoms of depression. Dilute two or three drops of them in five drops of grapeseed oil and it rub into the back of your hand, stomach or solar plexus; alternatively, drop it into a soothing bath. This may also be a good time to visit an aromatherapy practitioner, as the feelings of isolation that come from depression are often soothed by contact with others and a nurturing treatment such as an aromatherapy massage.

Diet

A disturbed sugar balance can also exacerbate depression, so make sure you eat a balanced diet and avoid stimulants that can give you mood and energy spikes. It may be tempting to reach for the chocolate, cigarettes or wine for comfort, but they will only add to the problem. Season food with marjoram and thyme for their antidepressant effects. Switch to teas such as mint, verbena and thyme to give you a lift and stop you from turning to stimulants such as tea and coffee. Wheatgerm is a great energizer so sprinkle it over your salads or cereals, and eat bromine-packed pears and apples for their soothing effect on the nervous system. In general, add more tryptophan-rich foods to your diet for their soothing properties (see page 52).

Supplements

5-HTP, a precursor to tryptophan that helps the body to produce serotonin (the body's happy chemical), is a very useful supplement. Exercise will also produce this hormone, so make sure you get outside and walk every day, even if is only for 20 minutes. Being in the daylight can also help with seasonal affective disorder (SAD) depression by providing you with much-needed vitamin D. Boosting your intake of omega 3 oils, B complex, vitamin C, vitamin E and ginseng will also improve your ability to cope with the stress of depression. If your diet is suffering from a loss of appetite or an inability or disinterest in cooking, make sure you take a good all-round multivitamin.

Herbal Help

St John's wort is a popular herbal alternative to prescribed antidepressants, but it can affect other conventional medicines used to treat illnesses such as asthma, heart problems and HIV. Anyone currently

RIGHT **Taking care of yourself through good diet and soothing, lifting herbal teas or supplements will improve your mood and sense of self-worth.**

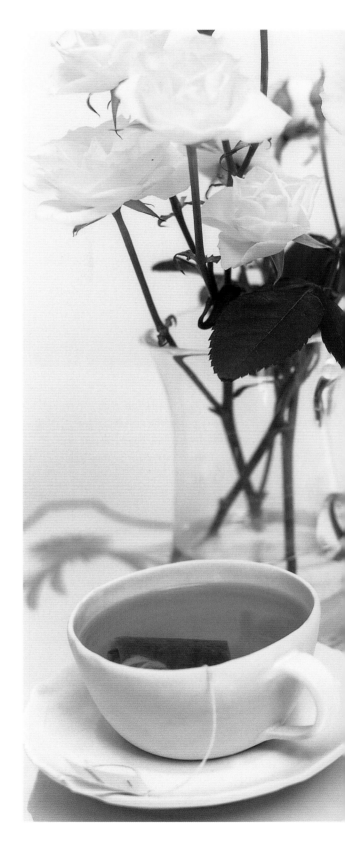

on medication must speak to his or her doctor about the suitability of taking this herb. Assuming all is well, St John's wort can be incredibly effective.

Homeopathy

Depending on the cause of your depression, or just your resulting feelings, you may find it helpful to try one of these remedies. Each works on a slightly different manifestation of the condition.

PULSATILLA

Good for those who are excessively weepy and tend to cry easily, but feel better after a cry.

NATRUM MUR

Good for those who cannot accept sympathy and tend to become introverted, shunning other people's company. They may find it hard to talk about their feelings or ask for help, and become irritable.

BELOW **Using several homeopathic treatments at once can help alleviate specific symptoms associated with your personal experience of depression.**

SEPIA

Can help those whose depression stems from a physical or mental exhaustion and who display feelings of apathy or indifference. They may feel weary and are easily offended. It is especially beneficial for men.

ARSENICUM ALBUM

Useful for helping those who wake in the night worrying about things and who berate themselves for their failure to meet their own exceptionally high standards.

LYCOPODIUM

This remedy is useful when there has been a loss of confidence, such as when a person's ability to cope with a job has been affected, making them forgetful and sensitive to criticism or contradiction. They may feel needy and dislike being on their own.

Flower Remedies

Bach Flower remedies can help rebalance some of the negative feelings associated with depression. Try using holly for alleviating anger, willow for bitterness and pine for guilt.

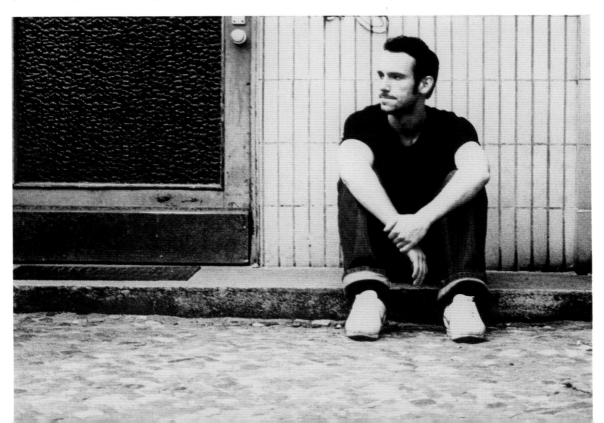

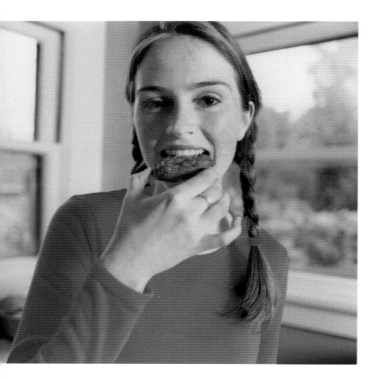

PERSISTENT FATIGUE

There are several reasons for the occurrence of persistent and chronic fatigue. As well as poor sleep, a diet lacking in nutrients can often be to blame. The two usually go hand in hand as we grab food on the go, especially sugar- and stimulant-crammed food to keep us going. The result of this kind of lifestyle is a body that is overloaded with toxins and that is hard to detoxify.

Common Symptoms

- Feeling weary
- Weepiness
- Feeling tired upon waking
- Falling asleep early

Aromatherapy

When you really need a perk, but can't take a break, geranium essential oil is a great pick-me-up. Mix 10 ml (2 tsp) of soya oil and five drops of geranium oil together, and massage it into the back of your neck, sinus area, back of the hands, temples and clockwise into the solar plexus, then lie flat, resting for five minutes.

Body Brushing

Dry body brushing your skin is a very hands-on way of getting your lymphatic fluid, which carries toxins out of the body and takes much-needed nutrients to the tissues, working at its best. As well as shaking off fatigue, it has the added bonus of helping prevent premature ageing. Using a firm, natural bristle brush (but not so firm that it scratches) work in large upward movements from the feet, up the front and backs of legs and including your buttocks. For the upper body, the action should be in circular motions towards the heart, in an up or down direction (be careful over any damaged or sensitive skin). Body brushing also improves your skin's tone and texture, getting rid of dead skin cells, and leaving the skin smoother and fresher looking.

Homeopathy

Kali. phosphorus can be used to treat weakness and tiredness, especially if it has been caused by worry, excitement or overwork.

Exercise

Gentle exercise will get the lymph drainage system moving. No matter how reluctant you feel about attempting it, even getting off the bus a stop earlier or walking rather than driving will give you a boost.

Diet

Eat little and often. Choose slow-release carbohydrates, such as porridge, and fresh fruit. Avoid all stimulants, such as tea, coffee, sugar, cigarettes, chocolate, cola drinks and alcohol.

Supplements

Vitamin C (1,000 mg) and an antioxidant complex will help your body detoxify. An antioxidant complex will help mop up the damaging toxins.

ABOVE **Making sure that your diet is rich in nutrients and high in energy is a good way of tackling fatigue. Avoid relying on chocolate or biscuits for an energy lift.**

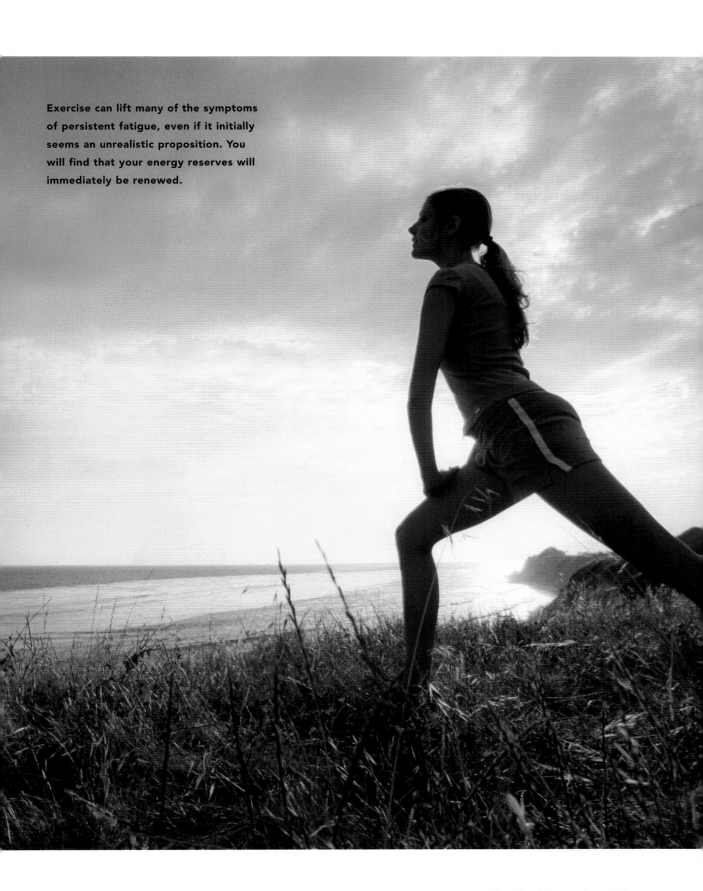

Exercise can lift many of the symptoms of persistent fatigue, even if it initially seems an unrealistic proposition. You will find that your energy reserves will immediately be renewed.

VANISHED LIBIDO

Exhausted new parents may have making more babies low on their list of priorities, but for many of us a missing sex drive can be a saddening and frustrating experience. A low libido can be due to hormone imbalance, depression or simply fatigue.

Common Symptoms

- A lack of interest in sex
- Avoiding physical intimacy with your partner

Your Environment

Make sure your bedroom is more 'boudoir' than dumping ground. It's hard to relax and feel sexy if you can't switch off from the pressures of the day because you can see them out of the corner of your eye. Take a look at pages 84–7 for some good ideas for getting back in the mood.

Diet

Increase your intake of seafood, wholegrain bread, green leafy vegetables, crumbly cheeses and lean meat. These all contain zinc, a lack of which can result in a low libido. Don't rely on alcohol to get you in the mood; it can cause impotence in men and make it difficult for many women to achieve orgasm.

Aromatherapy expert Daniele Ryman, in her book *Aromatherapy Bible*, recommends a glass of this basil aphrodisiac drink before meals to encourage your sex drive.

1 litre (1¾ pints) of red wine from Cahors
50 g (2 oz) of fresh basil leaves

Uncork the bottle of wine, pour a little out to make room for the basil leaves, push the leaves into the bottle and replace the cork. Leave for two days to mature in the dark, shaking from time to time.

Supplements

A zinc supplement can help if your diet is lacking.

BELOW **The loss of interest in sex that can result from exhaustion or depression can cause further stress in relationships.**

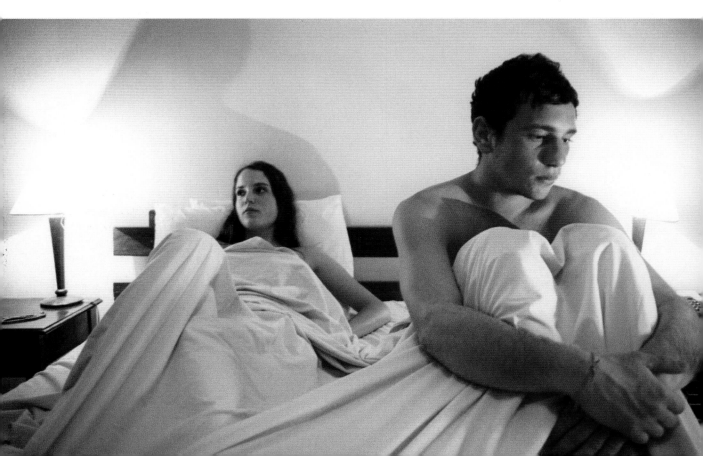

FEELING 'HUNGOVER' WHEN YOU WAKE UP

Even if you have been working on improving your sleeping patterns, you can occasionally wake with a muggy-headed sensation. This can be a result of the body still trying to work off a sleep deficit, over-sleeping or poor-quality sleep. It may also be that you are grinding your teeth, producing pressure in your jaw. Your dentist should be able to tell if this is happening and may be able to give you a mouthguard to help counteract it.

Common Symptoms
- Reluctance to get out of bed
- Feeling of not being sufficiently rested
- Irritability
- Lack of coordination
- Craving for stimulants, such as tea or coffee

Your Environment

Making sure your room is not too dark or too light is vital. Too much light in the room will result in a lack of melatonin production, which means you will have a lighter, more broken sleep. Too much darkness, on the other hand, means an over-production of melatonin that will leave you feeling as if you are being woken up in the middle of the night. Curtains that darken the room sufficiently to allow sleep, yet let the dawn's emergence become visible, are essential. If you cannot achieve both, try heavy curtains and a sunlight alarm clock that impersonates the dawn and lets the body start its natural production of cortisol to prepare it for the day ahead. Making sure you get up at the same time every day also helps the body to prepare for daytime demands.

Acupressure

This ancient system can pep you up in minutes. For quick relief, squeeze your ears quite firmly between your thumb and forefinger, starting with the lobes and going around the edge, holding each pinch a few seconds at a time. Alternatively, seek treatment with a practitioner.

Aromatherapy

Lemon oil will give you more energy, and an aromatherapy soap, such as grapefruit, will wake you up. If your poor sleep has been caused by catarrh or congestion, try inhaling essential oils before you go to bed to clear your sinuses. Cajuput, tea tree or geranium essential oils dropped into hot water to make vapours are all great for clearing the sinuses. The next morning, a bath with pepper or juniper oil will liven you up.

Diet

Cutting out dairy products can help stop the build-up of mucus caused by illness or poor congestion.

BAD BREATH

Occasional bad breath upon waking can have several causes. Breathing through the mouth, perhaps due to a cold or congestion, can be a cause, or it may be an oral health issue, such as tooth decay, saliva and mouth bacteria or gum infections. Bad breath can also be an indicator of other health problems, such as poor food digestion or lung and respiratory problems. Try over-the-counter mouthwashes and a visit to your dental hygienist. If these fail, consult a doctor.

Common Symptoms
- Pungent odour
- Unpleasant fuzziness in the mouth
- Discoloured tongue

Herbal Help

Make your own mouthwash from one drop of myrrh essential oil in a cup of cooled, boiled water. If you find the taste unpalatable, camomile, fennel, mint or thyme can be used instead.

Diet

Chewing parsley, thyme, tarragon, anise seeds or a cinnamon stick can all help. Take a note of your diet and see if there are any foods that cause you particular problems; spicy foods and garlic are often problematic.

Homeopathy

KALI. PHOSPHORUS
Should be used if the mouth is dry and the tongue is coated yellow/brown.

MERCURIUS SOLUBILIS
Should be used if you suffer from bad breath and a sore tongue, especially noticeable while chewing, accompanied by excessive thirst.

RECURRENT COLDS AND INFECTIONS

Lack of sleep is often accompanied by a general run-down sensation, making you feel even less resilient and in control. This is due to a depressed immune system, which struggles to fight off the infections that attack us every day. Regardless of external pressures, you really must try to prioritize sleep at this point. When your body shuts down non-essential functions, it concentrates on repair and maintenance.

Common Symptoms
- Increased frequency of coughs and colds
- Propensity to catch any bugs that seem to be circulating

Herbal Help
Replace your regular brew with cat's-claw tea with ginger, four times daily. Drinking an infusion of rose petals, or gargling with them, will help settle a cough that may be keeping you awake. Echinacea will shorten the length of a cold and help protect against the onset of new ones.

Diet
A good balanced diet should maintain your system, but too much protein can suppress vitamin B6, which is essential for recovery. Avoid saturated fat, as it can suppress immunity, whereas essential fats, those present in cold-pressed seed oil such as pumpkin or flax, can boost it. Watermelon juice, carrot soup and a snack of berries can all boost your immune system, too.

Supplements
For the immune system to function properly it needs vitamins A, B1, B2, B6, B12, folic acid, C and E, and the minerals iron, zinc, magnesium and selenium. A good-quality multivitamin should ensure you get all of these. If you still feel exhausted, take grapefruit seed and elderberry extract.

Homeopathy

ACONITE
A fast-acting homeopathy remedy that can ease feverishness, sore eyes and throat.

GELSEMIUM
Will help flu-like symptoms, such as chills, muscle aches and spasms, stuffed-up nose and a dry throat.

POOR SKIN

When lacking good-quality sleep, your skin can quickly indicate the stresses, and this is often exacerbated by a poor diet. A lack of sleep reduces your immunity, making you more prone to infections, including skin infections. The skin gains access to nutrients during the night and repairs any existing damage then, so poor sleep will disrupt this process. Your doctor may suggest topical steroid treatment creams for application directly to the problem skin areas.

Common Symptoms
- Spots, pimples and cold sores
- Sallow and dull appearance
- Flare-ups of conditions like psoriasis or acne

Skincare Routine
Make sure you cleanse, tone and moisturize your skin each morning and night to reduce the chance of any flare-ups. A good-quality night cream, loaded with antioxidants and vitamins, will help the skin in its repair work. Smokers should look for oxygen creams to help counteract the damage caused by smoking. For a quick boost, a gentle exfoliator will slough off dead skin and bring back a fresh glow.

To get the blood circulating, try this quick exercise. Stand with your legs two or three feet apart. Place your hands on your hips, bend from the waist out and down toward the floor, keeping your legs straight. Now place your palms on the floor and keep stretching gently downward. Slowly creep your hands forward for a bigger stretch and then breathe deeply for 10–15 breaths. Reverse your moves, bringing your hands back to your feet then up to your hips. Make sure you do all of this slowly so that you don't feel dizzy.

Diet

Strawberries, blueberries and raspberries are all very rich in vitamin C, which helps strengthen the collagen in the skin. They also have a high concentration of antiageing antioxidants.

Try blending these ingredients in a smoothie:

100 g (3½ oz) mixed berries
1 small banana
1 small pot of plain yogurt
150 ml (¼ pint) skimmed or soya milk.

Supplements

If cold sores are a persistent problem, try lysine supplements daily. An amino acid, lysine counteracts foods that can encourage cold sores.

BELOW **Poor skin tone and an increase in blemishes or skin complaints are signs of a body stressed through lack of good sleep or good nutrition.**

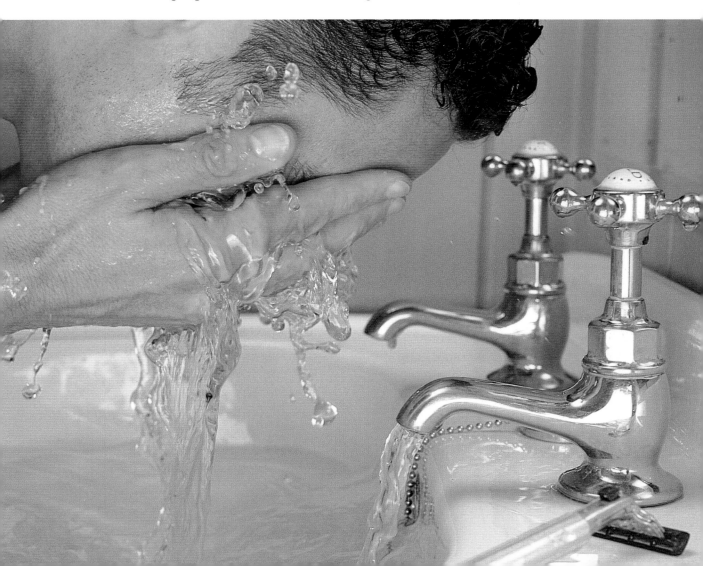

RECURRENT HEADACHES

Headaches, as anyone who frequently suffers from them will tell you, can come in many different forms. Try and write down the symptoms and times to see if there is a pattern. You may find that you have a headache after staring at your computer screen or when your blood sugar drops after a lunch on the go.

Common Symptoms

- Dull, throbbing pain around the head, neck, and temples and/or behind the eyes
- Feeling like a tight band is fixed around the head
- Sensitivity to light or noise

Aromatherapy

Effective in relieving headaches, aromatherapy is also a soothing treatment that can help with anxiety and tension that may be related to the headaches. Try blending the following:

2 drops of essential peppermint oil
3 drops of essential lavender oil
5 drops of eucalyptus oil.

Add to a cream or gel base and apply to the temples and the base of the neck. If these scents do not appeal, then try a single drop of basil, camomile, juniper (this also gives off a small amount of heat so is great for muscle tension in the neck), rosemary or clary sage in 5 ml (1 tsp) of grapeseed oil. This will bring relief when massaged onto the neck, temples or around the eyes (always be careful when putting any oils near your eyes).

Acupressure

Try this simple acupressure treatment on yourself, wherever you are. Press a finger into your eye sockets near the nose for a few seconds, several times. Alternatively, press the web of skin between your thumb and forefinger for two or three minutes (using the thumb and forefinger of your other hand). Swap hands and repeat.

Homeopathy

A good homeopathic remedy is gelsemium, especially for help with 'tight band' headaches. Acid phosphorus can help with headaches brought on by eye strain or tiredness.

Herbal Help

Lime flower, valerian or verbena will all help tension headaches.

Diet

Headaches are often due to low-level dehydration, so increasing your water intake should help – 2.5 litres (4¼ pints) is the recommended amount. Eat often and in small amounts so you avoid blood sugar crashes, making sure you choose something with a low glycaemic index (see page 50).

High-fibre foods can help cushion the mood swings that bring on headaches. Avoid acidic fruits, such as citrus fruits, as they can aggravate headaches and migraines; opt for pears instead.

Supplements

Vitamin C (1,000 mg) and vitamin B3 (100 mg) are especially effective at heading off migraines.

DARK CIRCLES AROUND THE EYES AND PUFFY EYELIDS

Often seen as a sign of a late night, dark circles around your eyes are, according to Chinese medicine, a sign of the body's inability to drain impurities. The purplish colour, along with puffiness, is the result of poor circulation in tiny blood vessels. The skin under the eyes is so thin that if the blood vessels are swollen, they show up very clearly and are a definite sign that you are not getting enough sleep. They can also simply be hereditary. A doctor may prescribe a vitamin A-derivative cream or refer you to a dermatologist for a prescription bleach cream. If you are going to indulge, set aside a few nights for the body to recover; it will make the areas around your eyes look much clearer.

Common Symptoms

- Dark patches under the eyes
- Dull texture to the skin
- Swollen lids

Skincare Routine

Dark circles under the eyes can be hidden, to some extent, with cosmetics. Select a concealer that is one shade lighter than your foundation. One with a pale yellow undertone will help hide blue- or grey-toned circles. A blue or mauve underbase masks brown-toned under-the-eye bags. Dab concealer under your eyes gently.

Eating well is good for general eye health and can help reduce the effects of poor sleep, such as dark circles and red eye. Vitamin A improves night vision and is found in dark green, leafy vegetables, carrots, spinach, broccoli, eggs, cheese and butter. Carotene allows the formation of visual purple in the eyes, which helps improve weak eyes. Good sources of carotene are carrots, broccoli, cabbage and peas. Vitamin B complex is excellent for reducing redness in eyes and it can also help eyes that are sensitive to light. Good food sources for vitamins B1, B2, B3, B6 and B12 are pasta, bread, milk, dark green

vegetables, tuna, nuts, mushrooms, avocados, bananas and liver.

Don't just eat the food though. Take slices of cucumber straight from the fridge, for its cooling and soothing effect, or use one small slice of potato. Put a slice under each eye and leave them for 20 minutes. This will firm the skin and constrict the blood vessels. Alcohol, smoking and late nights should also be avoided or minimized.

To improve the drainage from under the eye, use an under-eye cream made with plant or marine extracts or antioxidants such as vitamin C and soya, which get toxins moving and moisturize the delicate under-eye skin. Apply morning and night with a light tapping motion to stimulate circulation and prevent puffiness.

Herbal Help

Soothing eye pads placed on the eyelids help encourage drainage from this sensitive area. Use cotton make-up remover pads dipped in cooled camomile or green tea. Alternatively, try this mix using diluted euphrasia (eyebright herb) tincture:

30 ml (2 tbsps) euphrasia (eyebright)
2 cups of hot water
2 cotton pads.

Steep the herb in water for three minutes or until cooled. Strain, dip a cotton pad into the liquid and wipe the eyes.

Diet

Increase your water intake to help your body flush out the toxins. Reduce salt, which can inflate eye bags, and avoid caffeine, a diuretic that will counteract the effect of the water.

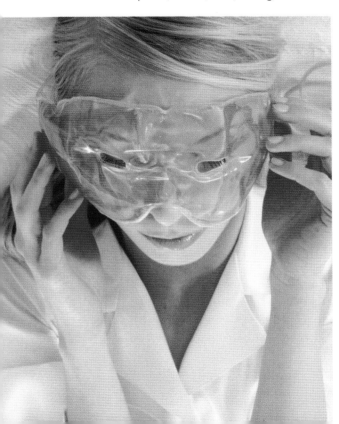

LEFT **Puffy skin and dark eye bags are an immediate giveaway that you have been burning the candle at both ends; a cool compress over the eyes will provide relief almost instantly.**

JET LAG

The frequency of air travel now means that jet lag is a familiar experience for many of us, but is no less draining. Over-the-counter or prescribed sleeping tablets are often used to force the body to fit in with new night-time schedules, and caffeine tablets to prevent the onset of sleep are also used.

Common Symptoms

- Disorientation
- Exhaustion
- Stomach upsets
- Nausea
- Fatigue
- Dehydration

Aromatherapy

Use 2–3 drops of essential oil, such as cypress or rosemary, in 15 ml (1 tbsp) of grapeseed or soya oil, and massage it into the soles of the feet to promote circulation and prevent leg cramps and swollen ankles.

Massage

If you are trapped in a window seat, try to do foot exercises. Squeeze your toes together, hold for a count of five, and then release. Do this 10–15 times in each session. If you need to stay awake when you arrive, rub ten drops of lavender oil onto your torso and immediately follow it with a shower. To sleep, take a bath with three drops of geranium oil added.

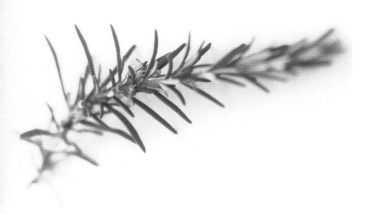

Homeopathy

Cocculus will help a headache brought on by travel, especially headaches that feel much worse when you are lying down.

Diet

During the flight, try to eat only citrus fruits. Increase your intake of still water (fizzy water can add to the feeling of being swollen and bloated) and avoid all dehydrating tea, coffee and alcohol.

Flower Remedies

Start taking a Bach Flower remedy combination a couple of days before the flight and continue it while you are flying and after, until all the symptoms have gone.

OLIVE

Helps you over the physical exhaustion of travelling and being on the move.

WALNUT

Helps you to adjust to a new time zone and place.

IMPATIENS

Stops you from getting impatient while sitting in a plane for several hours.

Supplements

Vitamin B complex can help your body cope with the stress of flying and adjust more quickly to the new time zone.

RIGHT **Jet lag is the conflict between our internal clock and the external reality; making the effort to stay awake when it's daylight will make the transition easier.**

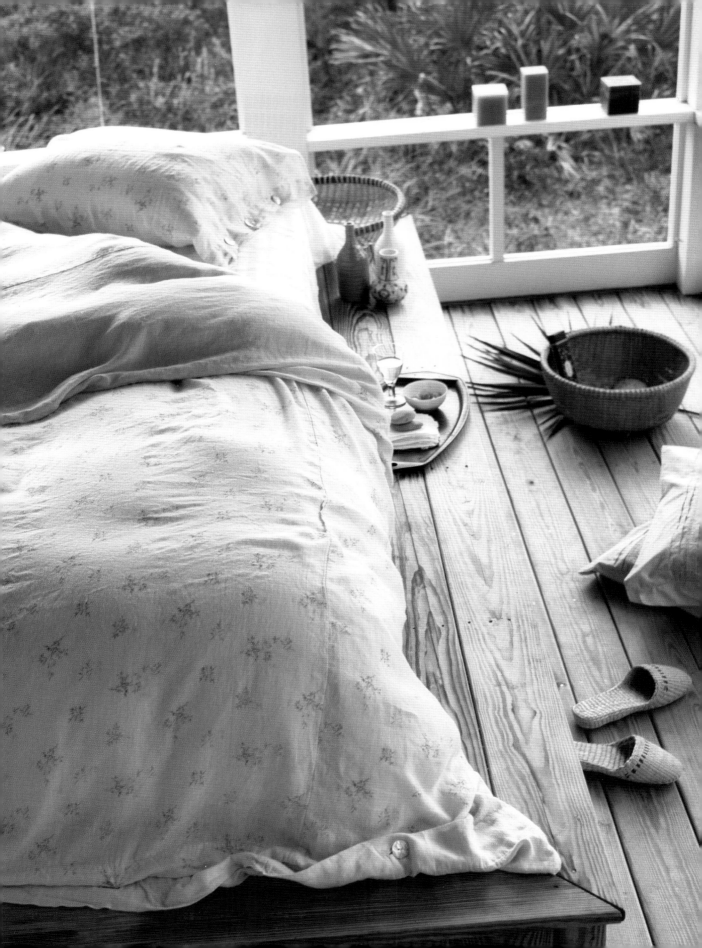

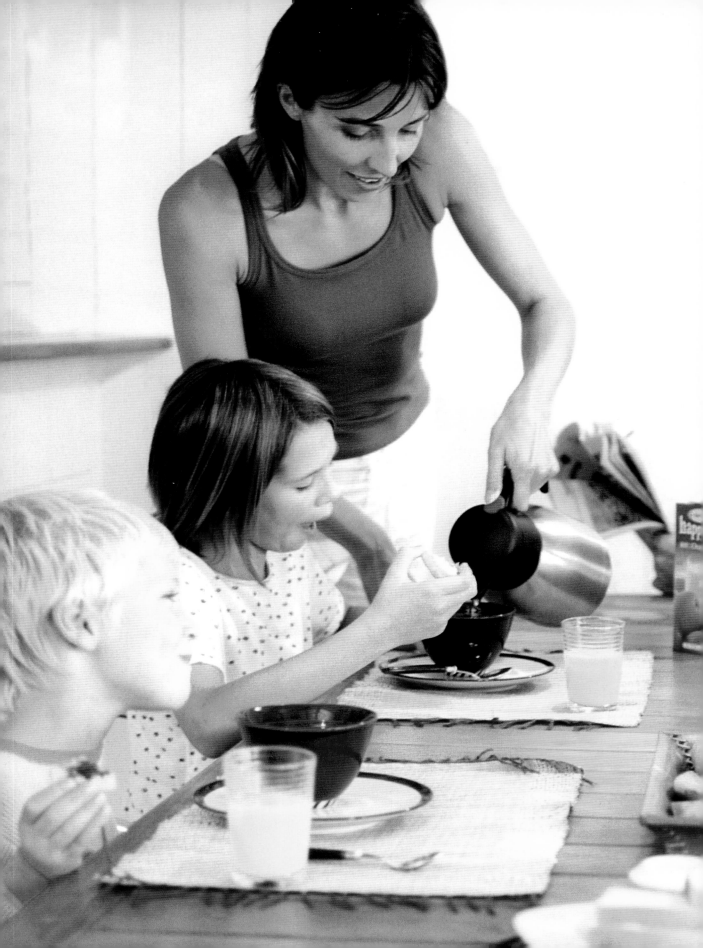

7 Family Sleep Health

A S WITH ALL OTHER ASPECTS OF LIFE, our relationship to and experience of sleep changes throughout our lifetime, which is why we might find previously tried-and-tested methods for restoring good sleep patterns fail us.

Like the frustrated parent who drags a 'slovenly' teenager out of bed, worrying that they are sleeping their life away, we can accidentally work against the body's biological needs through a lack of understanding; teenagers' developing brains and bodies actually need those extra hours, and they are not being lazy, no matter what the parent might think. When we consider that we often ignore our own chronic fatigue by refusing to cut down on work or social commitments, it's easy to see where the misunderstandings come from. Taking time out to examine the patterns and needs of those around us can greatly improve our tolerance, and our effectiveness at achieving satisfying slumber for the whole family.

Every family member may be unique in their sleep requirements, circadian rhythm and the amount of sleep they need for their specific stage in life. When we understand this, our waking hours together with our family members can be less fraught with exhaustion and tension, too – snappy, grumpy breakfasts can be a thing of the past.

LEFT **Harmonious and happy family breakfasts are often achieved after a good night's sleep.**

NEWBORNS AND BABIES

Our relationship with sleep begins long before we are even aware of its existence (or even our own). A foetus spends a great deal of time asleep, between about 16 to 20 hours out of 24, much of which is thought to be spent in the REM stage. Even our birth is influenced heavily by sleep; sleep expert William C Dement recorded the fact that mothers often go into labour at night, which is thought to be designed to make sure that the birth takes place in a safe home environment.

Once the baby has joined us on the 'outside', it has only two stages of sleep, spending about 50 per cent, or eight hours, in REM and the rest in non-REM. You can usually tell which sleep stage a baby is in. With adults, REM sleep is accompanied by paralysis so we don't imagine we are flying and launch ourselves from the bedroom window, but in newborn infants, this mechanism has yet to develop, so you can observe them twitching and wriggling through their dreams. Their non-REM sleep is entirely passive and still. A smaller baby often needs more sleep than larger babies of the same age.

It takes several weeks for newborns to sleep in any kind of solid patterns or for any length of time. In the initial stages, parents seem summoned at all hours by cries in no obvious pattern, and the parents lose at least two hours of sleep a night for the first five months (after the first year, on average, a parent is losing only an hour a night of sleep). At about eight weeks the child seems to start displaying some sensitivity to day and night, and the sleep periods will begin to be consolidated into longer stretches at night-time. By about four to six weeks the baby has begun to develop a circadian rhythm.

By six months, most infants are sleeping from 12 to 14 hours a day in a solid block with some naps, and the amount of time spent dreaming has dropped to the adult quota of 25 per cent. Although many parents can testify that children often still awaken during the night.

Happy Families

Parents should try to create a sleep plan that helps them cope with a newborn. Napping when the baby sleeps (in order to chip away at their own sleep deficit), working out who will take care of which tasks and making sure they support their own wellbeing with good-quality herbal and vitamin supplements (should their attention to their diets prove haphazard), are all essential at easing this initial period of stress. In the current climate, often both parents work and require enough rest to function in their daily tasks, and they'll both want to be in top form to be able to care for their child well. How to best provide for the needs of the whole family is always in constant debate, but research does show some interesting results for finding the best solution for everyone.

Helping Newborns Sleep

Studies have shown that babies who are breastfed spend more time in deep sleep with a lower pulse rate, compared with bottle-fed babies. Of course, many factors are involved when faced with the issue of feeding, so breastfeeding is not always a possible choice for the parent. However, parents can help the development of the circadian rhythm in a child by using light cues; a bright room in the morning and a dim one at night helps as does a

regular feeding schedule (small bellies mean that they need a new feed every four to five hours). Always avoid unnecessary stimulation such as turning on bright overhead lights, playing games or chatting away during the evening hours; it might relieve the tedium for you, but it will drag a baby even further into the waking world and inhibit a swift return to slumber.

If your newborn is having serious problems sleeping, you may want to consult a doctor to see if an allergy to the environment, or even the type of milk you are using, exists. Another major problem is colic. Occurring as frequently as one in every five babies, this condition has definite symptoms, but the cause is still not known, although it is thought to be connected to delayed development in the bowel. As night-time approaches, children with colic often can have recurring agitated crying and screaming attacks, which can last for hours at a time, and they can frequently reawaken during the night and cannot seem to be comforted. Fortunately, most babies outgrow colic by four months (although children who have suffered from colic are more likely to suffer from sleep disturbances later in childhood).

Three to Six Months

A child that falls asleep on its own is more likely to go back to sleep on its own if it wakes during the night. Placing a drowsy child in a cot will also help the child feel comfortable drifting off in that environment, rather than relying on parents' soothing. Your child may also be teething at this age; a good trick is to keep a cloth under your baby's head while it sleeps, to catch the excessive drool caused by this process. That way you can make a swift change during the night, swapping cloths rather than the whole sheet and cutting down on the disturbance.

RIGHT **Understanding your child's sleep development makes coping with restless nights much easier to bear.**

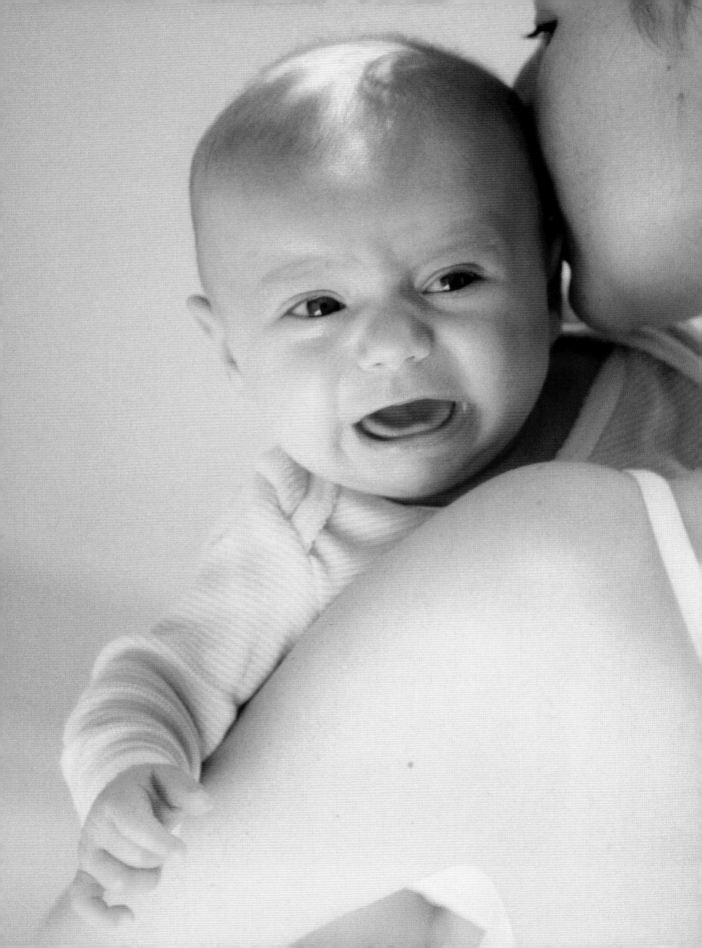

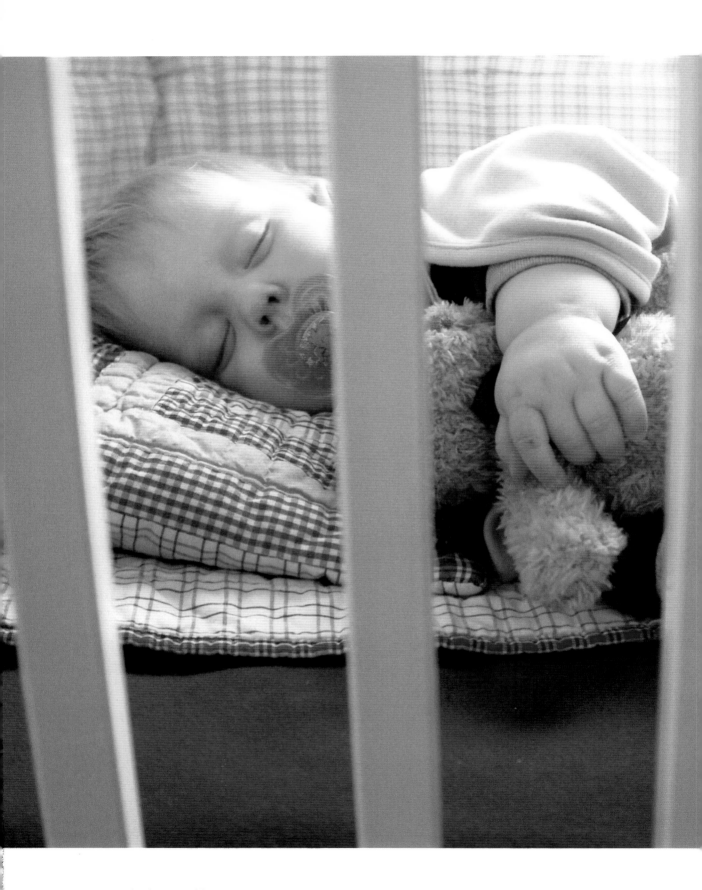

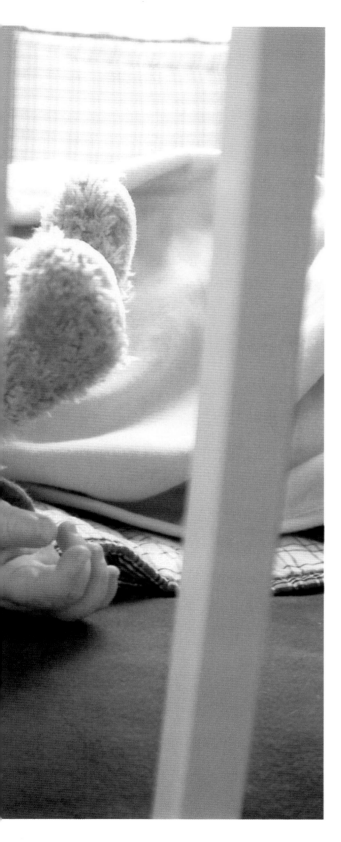

Six Months to Toddler

A child that is six months old should sleep about 11 hours a night, with a substantial nap during the day. This is the time that many parents want to implement a set routine. Don't give a child too many 'conditions' for sleep if you want them to achieve a 'return to rest' more easily; if they associate a certain combination of toys, songs, milk or rocking in the arms of a parent as necessary for achieving slumber, it will become impossible for them to do without these aids.

The most famous and widely used technique is the Ferber Method. This was devised by Richard Ferber of the Boston Children's Hospital in the 1970s. His work was based on the idea that we are not born with the ability to soothe ourselves back to sleep after a night-time awakening, but must learn it as a skill. Parents who concur with Ferber begin the process when a chid is roughly six months old, at a stage when they are thought to be physically and emotionally able to cope. (At this age a child should not need a night-time feed.) When a child awakens, the parent is instructed to enter the room and verbally comfort the child, but offers no physical soothing, then leaves the room, regardless of whether or not the child is still crying. If the child still cries, the parent returns five minutes later and repeats the process. Next time, the parent waits 10, then 15 minutes. On the first night, the longest wait period is 15 minutes for any crying session. The following night, the parents add five minutes onto any waiting time; so the periods are 10, 15 and 20 minutes. This continues over a period of several nights, usually two or three, by which time the child should be able to self soothe. Although hard on the heartstrings and ears of the parents, for many families it can be a truly productive exercise. Ferber's theory is expounded in his book *Solve*

LEFT As babies become toddlers, creating a good sleep system becomes essential in terms of the whole family getting enough sleep.

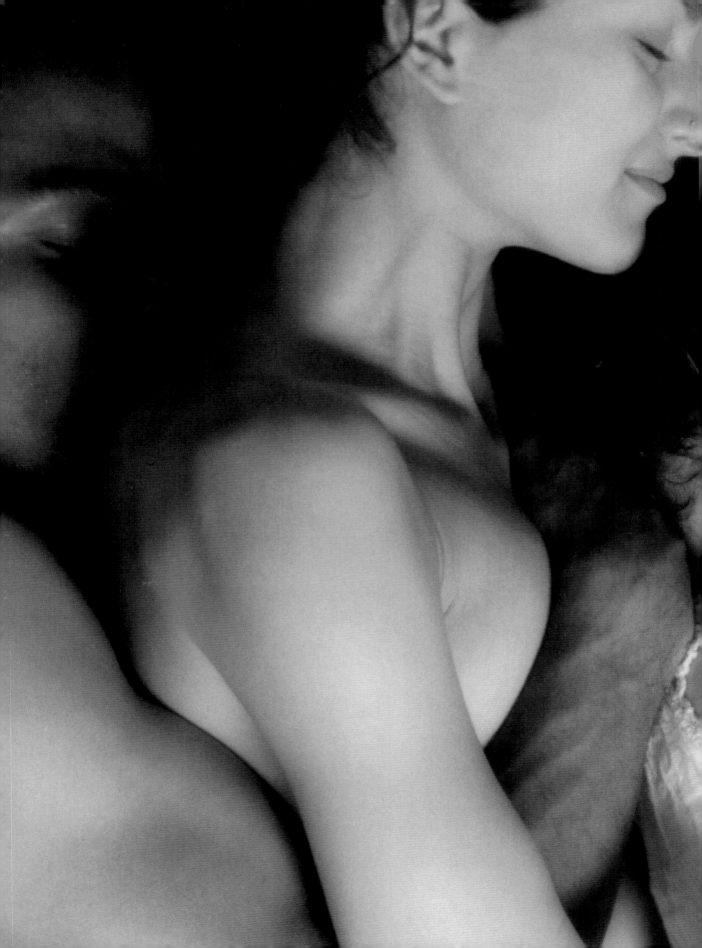

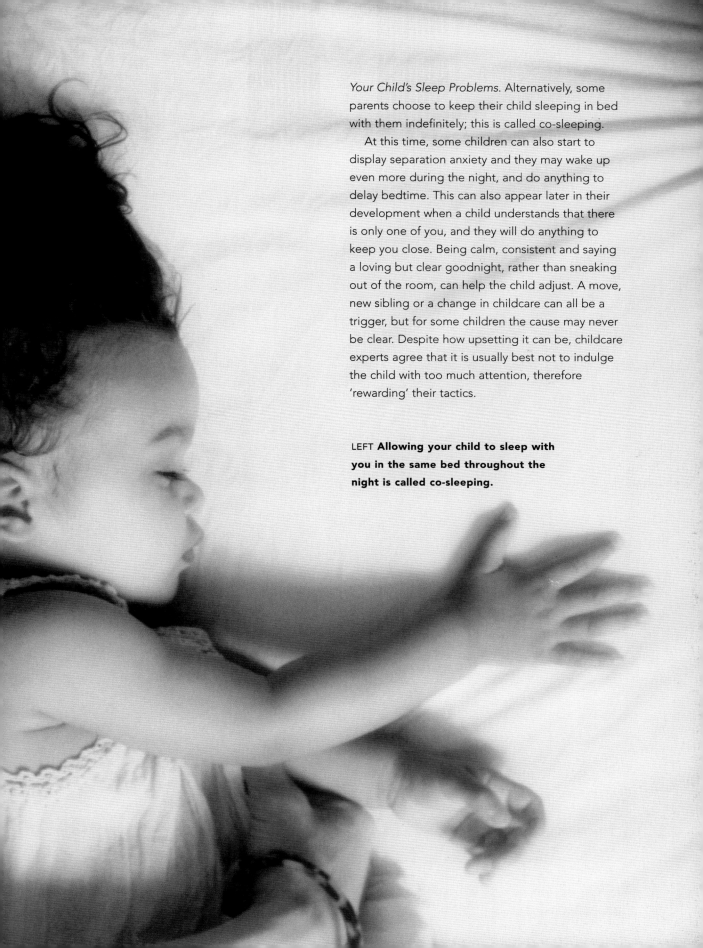

Your Child's Sleep Problems. Alternatively, some parents choose to keep their child sleeping in bed with them indefinitely; this is called co-sleeping.

At this time, some children can also start to display separation anxiety and they may wake up even more during the night, and do anything to delay bedtime. This can also appear later in their development when a child understands that there is only one of you, and they will do anything to keep you close. Being calm, consistent and saying a loving but clear goodnight, rather than sneaking out of the room, can help the child adjust. A move, new sibling or a change in childcare can all be a trigger, but for some children the cause may never be clear. Despite how upsetting it can be, childcare experts agree that it is usually best not to indulge the child with too much attention, therefore 'rewarding' their tactics.

LEFT **Allowing your child to sleep with you in the same bed throughout the night is called co-sleeping.**

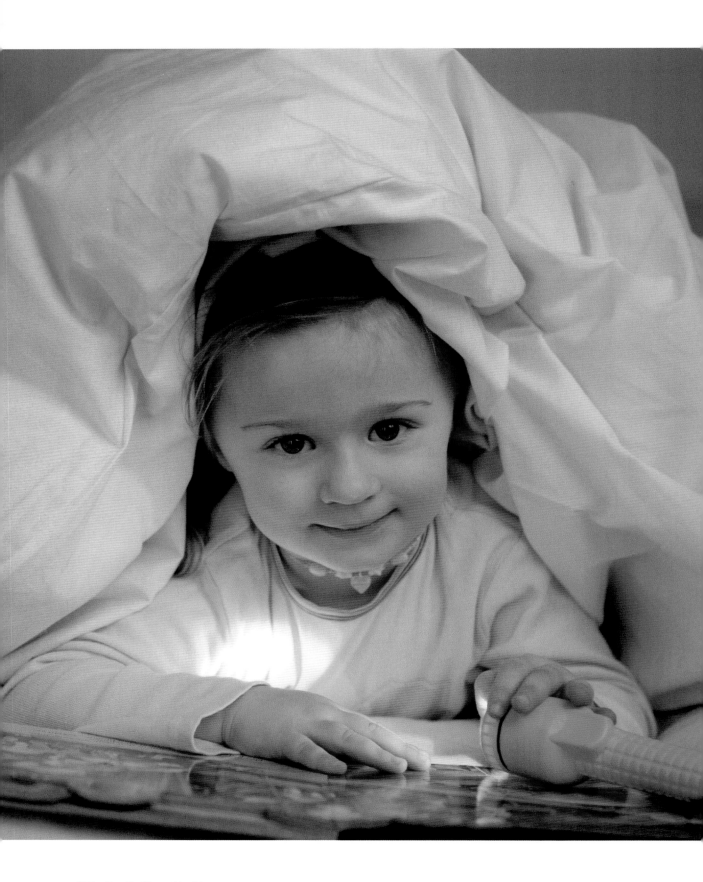

Bad Dreams and Night Terrors

For some children bad dreams and night terrors can become a problem. A night terror (also known as a parasomnia, Latin for 'near sleep', and associated with deep REM sleep) will find a child waking in the night screaming or shouting as if they are awake, although they will quickly go back to sleep and have no recollection of the experience the following day. Sleepwalking is also part of this category. Although it can be scary to witness, your child is not suffering and is actually sleeping through it. Most children grow out of it by the age of seven.

Nightmares occur mainly during REM sleep. Children suffer from them more than adults, and can be very distressed by them, especially as they may be unable to distinguish between reality and the dream. Many children grow out of them by adolescence, but a recurring nightmare could be a sign of stress or anxiety. Nightmares are commonplace when a house move, divorce or other major change has occurred.

LEFT Discussing bad dreams can help children to deal with their fears.

Advice for Nightmares

- Offer comfort, but do not overstimulate the child, and encourage them to get back to sleep as quickly as possible.
- Younger children who can't understand the concept of dreaming may need a cuddle and soothing voice. Older children should be encouraged to talk it through so you can dispel their fears.
- A night-light may help with fear of the dark, allowing them to soothe themselves back to sleep.
- With a recurring nightmare, an older child may benefit from talking the dream through during the day, then encouraged to change the ending to something more comforting or benign. This can actually help change the sequence of events the next time the dream is revisited.
- Avoid overstimulating television shows and books before bed.

BELOW **Soft night-lights can help banish frightening dark corners without disturbing their melatonin balance.**

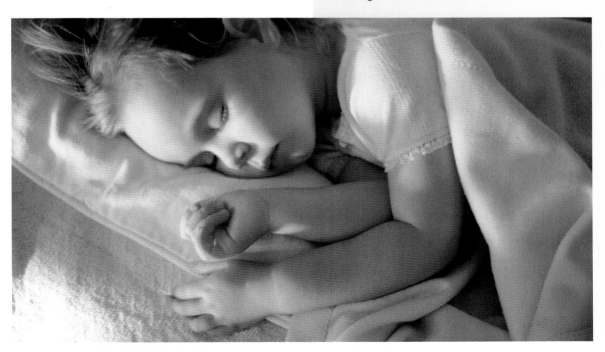

Devising a Bedtime Routine

Establishing a soothing sleep routine as early as possible is essential. The same events, such as bathing and stories, carried out in the same order every night, are a clear signal to a child that bedtime approaches, allowing them to naturally wind down. It is important that children of different ages have different bed times; try not to let the younger child's bedtime drift towards that of an older sibling. A good incentive should be that research shows that tired children underperform at school, are more likely to get into trouble and are more temperamental. Winning a battle at this time could save you from several the next day.

This simple routine can be used to easily guide your child from the transition of a fun-packed day to a restful night's sleep. Make sure the room is quiet and at a comfortable temperature 18°C (65 °F) is optimum). A night-light will comfort, but also allow you to attend any night-time awakenings without switching on a more powerful light. Make sure you don't allow the child to watch television up until the time you expect them to go to bed; they won't be able to make the transition from stimulation to rest that quickly. And avoid the temptation to put a TV in their room; this can send them mixed messages about what the bedroom is for – they need to see it as a place to rest.

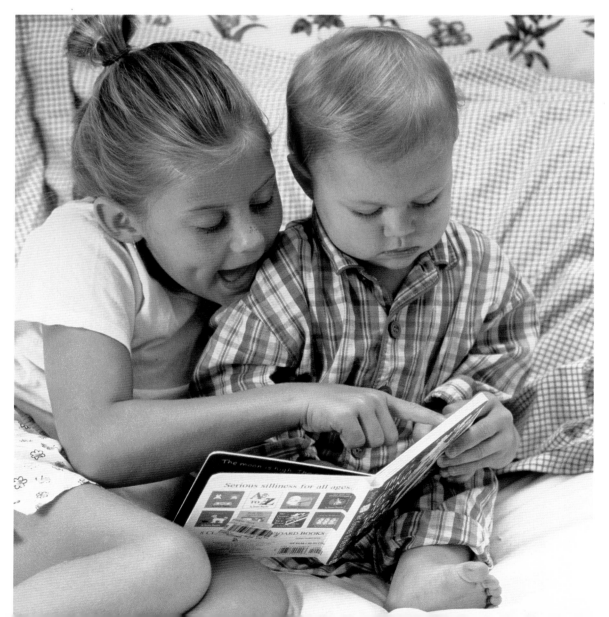

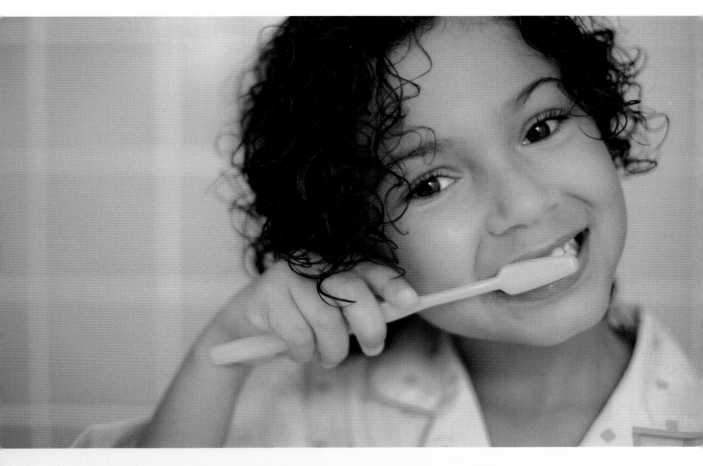

Establishing a Bedtime Routine

• Make bedtime the same time every night, alerting your child, or children, 30 minutes and then 10 minutes beforehand.

• Give your child a light snack, avoiding sugar or anything hard to digest. Don't give your baby or toddler a bottle (breast milk, formula, or any sugar-containing drink) to help him or her fall asleep. This can cause 'baby bottle tooth decay' because the fluids tend to pool in the baby's mouth.

• A warm bath will help lower your child's temperature, making them drowsy.

LEFT **Older siblings can read to younger ones in preparation for sleep. This will help both children settle into the routine.**

ABOVE **A good night-time routine helps children to wind down before bed and prepares them for sleep.**

• Put them in warm pyjamas after their bath so they feel cozy and comforted.

• Brush teeth.

• Read a story, but agree a maximum number, such as a two-book limit.

• Anticipate your child's last-minute requests, such as for a drink of water or a night-light, and incorporate them into the routine.

• Tuck your child into their beds, to promote a feeling of security and comfort.

• Say goodnight, tell him or her you'll be back to check on them in five minutes, and leave. They should be asleep by the time you return.

SCHOOL-AGE CHILDREN AND PRETEENS

Children ages 8 to 12 need a little over nine hours a night. A child at this age shouldn't need a daytime nap; in fact, children of this age should enjoy the ideal mix of total alertness and high energy during the day and a full, deep nourishing sleep at night. If your child does seem drowsy, try the Sleep Latency Test on page 18. Like adults, some children need more rest that others and identifying this will help you set a relevant bedtime.

Overtired children often exhibit exhaustion by excessive energy, grouchiness and tantrums. Some sleep experts, such as William C Dement who has created the esteemed Sleep Center at Stanford University, California, and launched the American Sleep Disorders Association, believes that some cases of ADHD (Attention Deficit Hyperactivity Disorder) are misdiagnosed; these children are simply excessively tired, and this manifests itself in a very similar way to ADHD.

A common behavioural disorder, children with ADHD act without thinking, find it difficult to focus or pay attention and are hyperactive. Boys are about three times more likely than girls to suffer from it. It can affect a child's family relationships and those with society in general, although improved understanding and treatment can provide great results. Treatment usually takes the form of medication and behavioural therapy. A doctor will need to diagnose the child with having the syndrome, and may make a referral to a neurologist, psychologist or psychiatrist. Many children can be fidgety or lack focus, but a child with ADHD displays these symptoms constantly and has problems controlling their behaviour without professional help. A child who has recently experienced a house move, separation of parents or other emotional disturbance may exhibit similar symptoms, but these should be temporary. Children with ADHD may also suffer from difficulties such as anxiety, and about half of all children with ADHD also have a specific learning disability such as dyslexia, which can add to their frustrations.

There are two main categories of ADHD, although a child may exhibit symptoms from both of them. Those with the 'inattentive' type may find it difficult to pay attention to details or they may produce sloppy schoolwork. They might find it difficult to follow instructions, be forgetful or seem distracted.

A 'hyperactive-impulsive' type can often be found fidgeting, always running or climbing, talking excessively and often interrupting others. It is important that these children are shown understanding and are diagnosed correctly in order to to help manage their symptoms. Children who do suffer from ADHD can experience a worsening of their symptoms if they don't get enough sleep.

Bedwetting

The American Academy of Child and Adolescent Psychiatry suggests that 15 per cent of three year olds wet the bed, which is also known as 'nocturnal enuresis'. Boys are more prone to do it than girls, and the problem can be a result of late development in bladder control, constipation or increased urine production. It is often hereditary. One way of controlling the problem is for the child to wear an alarm in their underwear that triggers as soon as the child begins to urinate – this can help train them to wake up. Plastic under the base sheet and on top of the mattress can help contain the mess if an accident occurs.

Limiting fluids, encouraging urination before bed and waking them in the night for a toilet trip will also help curb the problem. The most important thing is to avoid making the child ashamed as the child may become more anxious, which leads to broken sleep. No child wants to wake up in a cold, wet bed, so reassurance is key; almost all kids grow out of it relatively quickly. For persistent cases, seek help from a healthcare professional.

RIGHT **Nine hours' sleep is essential for ensuring that your preteens are bouncing and full of energy the next day.**

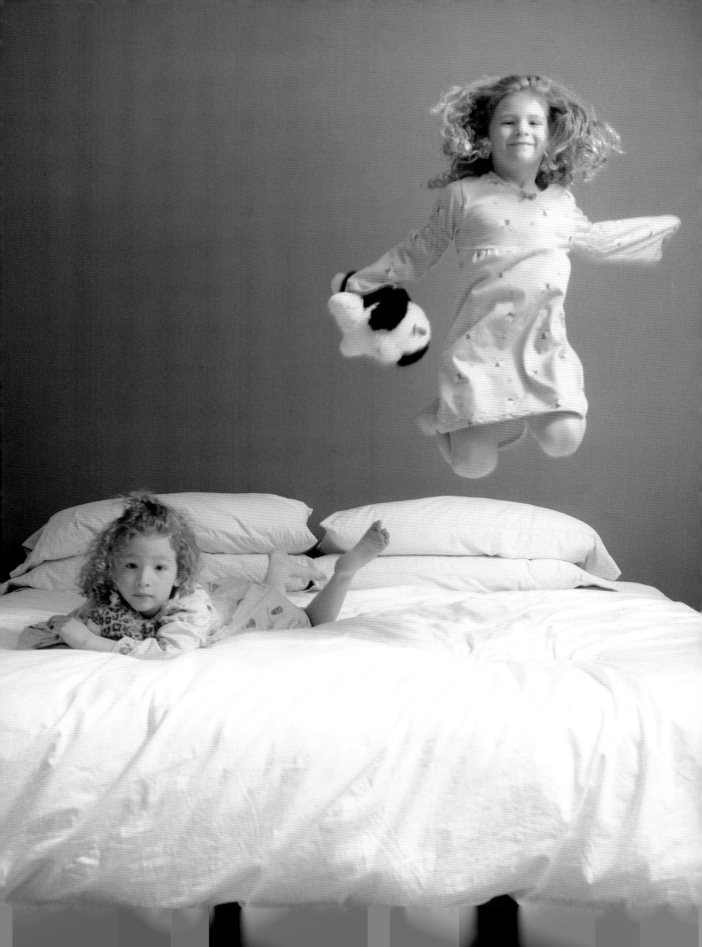

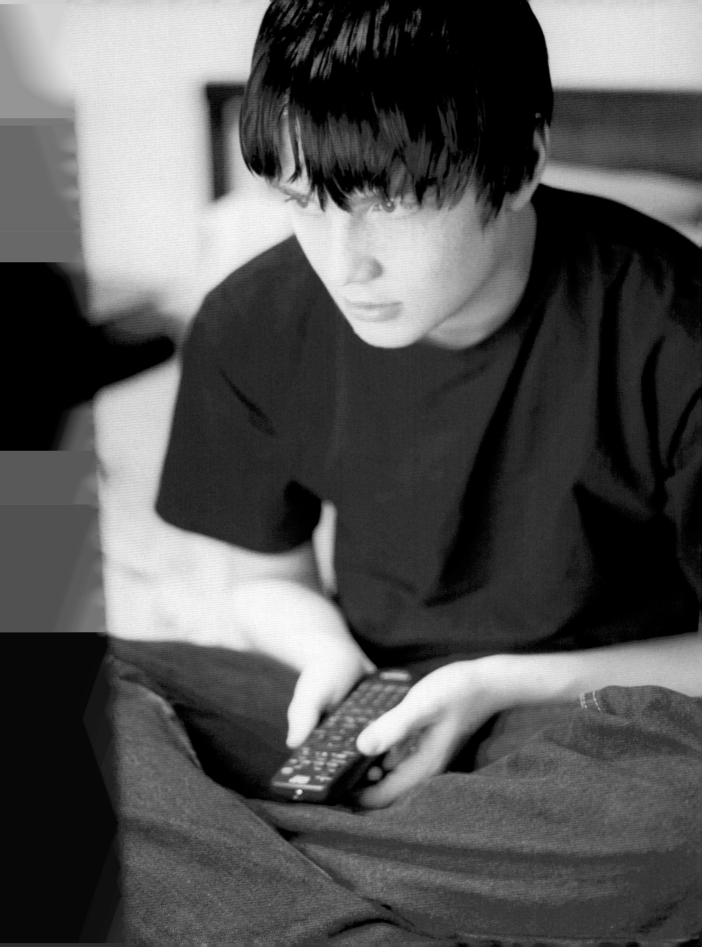

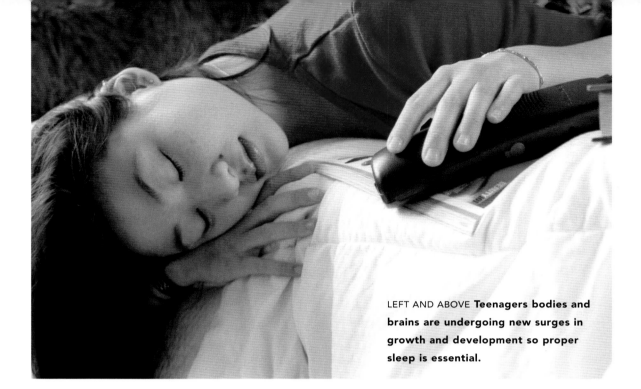

LEFT AND ABOVE **Teenagers bodies and brains are undergoing new surges in growth and development so proper sleep is essential.**

TEENAGERS

When it comes to sleep patterns, teenagers are often the most maligned of family members, with their desire to stay up all night and in bed all day, usually with important exams and commitments looming (which worried parents feel may dictate their whole future). In reality, adolescents need about 8 to 9½ hours of sleep per night, with this amount increasing as they make their way through their teens. But part-time jobs, homework and maintaining their ever-important social network eats into those essential hours. A bad-tempered, argumentative teenager will only become more difficult operating with a sleep deficit. Lack of focus, tolerance and comprehension can all affect their performance at school and a lack of sleep has been linked with increased outbursts of aggression and substance abuse.

Adolescents also experience a change in their sleep patterns in that their bodies want to stay up late, which often leads to them trying to catch up on sleep at the weekend. This is not purely designed to irritate parents; a shift in the circadian rhythm occurs at this time, making them stay up later. Although teenagers tend to be 'owls', by their thirties many become 'larks' (see page 17).

Hormones are making radical changes to the teenage body, with the cerebral cortex undergoing development, such as creating a sudden interest in the opposite sex. The growth hormone that generates puberty is also mostly released at night during sleep, making it vital they rest.

Ideally, a teenager would go to bed at the same time every night and wake up at the same time every morning, allowing for at least 8 to 9 hours of sleep. It may seem impossible to legislate for your teenager's behaviour, but trusting them to be in charge of their own sleep patterns may not be the best solution. Encouraging a consistent waking time, explaining how lack of sleep effects mood and discouraging stimulants such as late-night TV, computer games, caffeine drinks and sugar will all help them see sleep as an essential part of wellbeing. In the same way that removing gadgets and distractions from an adult room helps make it a restful environment, do the same for the teenager, making sure these temptations aren't part of their sleep space (see also page 69). A mind struggling to sleep will be too tempted to switch on the internet and while away the hours if it is clearly in view. Instilling in them the value of (and respect for) sleep can affect the quality of the rest of their lives.

THE WOMEN IN OUR LIVES: MOTHERS, DAUGHTERS, SISTERS

A woman's hormonal cycle will affect the quality of her sleep and the sleep of those around her throughout her life. The menstruation cycle, as any woman can tell you, can make her incredibly tired, whether before, during or just after her period. The American National Sleep Foundation released a poll that shows women's sleep quality is vastly affected by their cycle, with 71 per cent of women reporting that cramping, bloating, headaches and tender breasts disrupted their sleep during their period. Hormones causing changes in body temperature can also make sleep difficult.

Pregnancy has a huge affect on the way women sleep. In the same poll, 79 per cent reported more sleep disturbances at this time, and had an increased frequency of daytime sleepiness. The inability to get comfortable, the need to urinate more often and a kicking baby with no sense of the circadian rhythm can all add up to a restless night. Scientist Paul Martin records that pregnant women

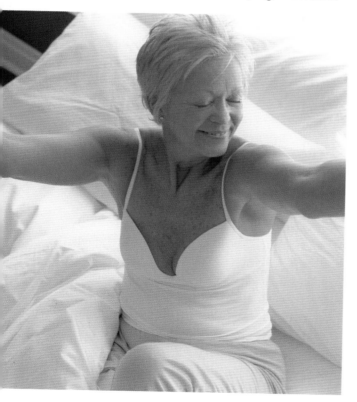

get only 5 per cent slow-wave sleep a night, compared to the average 25 per cent slow-wave sleep in normal adult sleep. Women also experience more dream sleep. A partner may be surprised to find that the woman suddenly becomes a snorer, which can have serious health implications for both mother and child, such as increased tendency to high blood pressure and pre-eclampsia. A doctor's advice should be sought immediately as help, such as special breathing masks, can relieve symptoms quickly.

Insomnia is often regarded as a key effect of menopause, which most women begin at around 50 years of age. Hot flashes, increased need to urinate, disordered breathing, mood disorders and other hormone-related changes all diminish good quality sleep. Oestrogen-replacement therapy and hormone-replacement therapy can help relieve symptoms in women, which tend to last a year but in some cases can last up to five, although there have been health concerns regarding their use (such as increased risk of breast cancer). Oestrogen is very effective for women suffering from menopausal insomnia, reducing the time it takes to fall asleep and decreasing the number of night-time awakenings. Some women prefer to use nutritional supplements such as calcium, vitamin D, soy products (which contain phytoestrogen, a plant compound similar to oestrogen), evening primrose oil, black cohosh and ginseng.

When experiencing menopause, or supporting someone who is, it is important to eat healthy meals, avoiding spicy or acidic foods that can trigger hot flashes. Keep the bedroom well ventilated and cool, and get professional help with anxiety or depression, which are treatable symptoms and do not have to be suffered quietly. Relaxation techniques, such as those on pages 80–4, can help reduce tension.

LEFT AND RIGHT **Throughout womens' lives, hormones play a large part in their quality of sleep.**

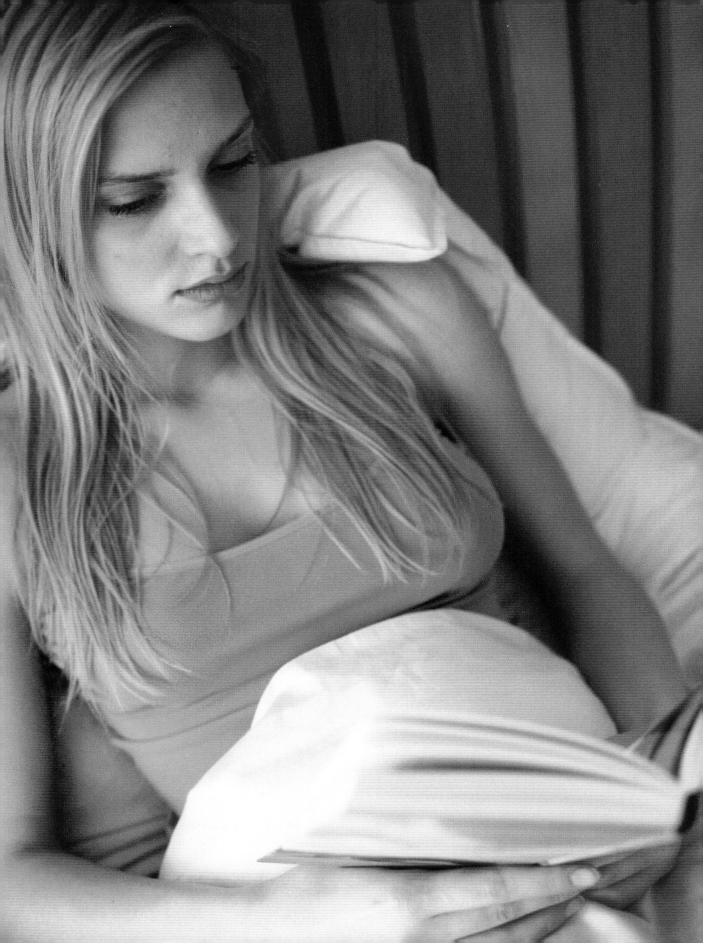

MIDDLE AGE AND PARTNER SLEEP

Although many of us will sleep with a partner at different stages of our lives, it is in middle age that most of us find this particular experience most challenging. The manifold pressures exerted upon us in middle age, from children, elderly parents, work and social responsibilities plus health challenges, all come at a time when we probably need our sleep most. Middle-aged and elderly women suffer the most from insomnia, and it's easy to understand why. Worry, an increase in snoring and sleep apnoea in partners, and the effects of menopause can all erode precious slumber.

Middle-aged people average seven hours per night, a gradual reduction of the requirement a person in their 20s needs. Middle-age weight gain can also increase the narrowing of the throat, which increases the chance and severity of snoring in both sexes. Sharing a bed with a partner means that whatever sleep challenges they may be facing, you will, too. You may simply be an owl and your partner a lark (see page 17), which can make your schedules difficult to reconcile (although with age we all drift towards lark tendencies). Understanding that neither partner is wilfully trying to be difficult, but rather that it is simply a predisposition, can help ease tensions.

Reliving the Tension

The best way to tackle such problems is to set aside fear of offending each other and be frank. Talk through the challenges you may now face: the following is a suggestion of possible solutions.

• Snoring is not a state that needs to be accepted by either party; through exercise, cutting back on alcohol and smoking and adopting a sensible diet, symptoms can be greatly relieved. As much as 99 per cent of cases can be treated.

• Women tend to get colder at night than men; duvets that are warmer on one half than the other are available, or use separate coverings.

• Couples, especially younger ones, tend to move in a synchronized way during the night, but older couples can become less in tune. Explore the possibility of buying a bigger bed with a mattress division (so you effectively each have your own mattress), which will allow you both to move freely without disturbing your partner.

• Illnesses, such as fybromalgia, or conditions like menopause, can also make sleep difficult, as can the medication that accompanies them. Be prepared to return to your doctor and discuss alternatives. You may have been given a convenient popular medication, but be better suited to an alternative.

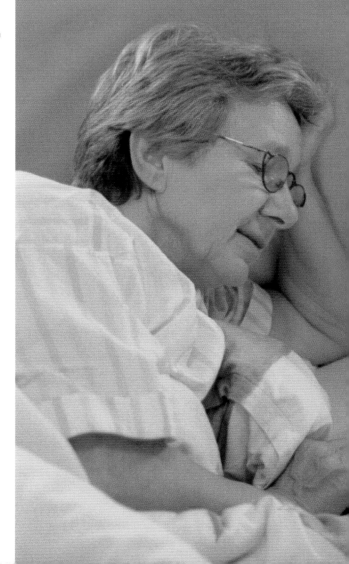

• Busy schedules and stress can eat into sleep through worrying. Write down all your concerns and schedule challenges and see what you can practically address, and what are just late-night fears. As well as helping you feel more in control, this will allow you to see if you have real room for practical improvement (such as a redistribution of chores) or have anxiety and relaxation issues.

• Make changes work. Some changes, such as the tendency towards 'larkness' and the reduction of hours needed to sleep, are a natural part of ageing. Perhaps the best way to deal with these changes is through acceptance; changing a schedule to take advantage of the peaceful morning hours to work or do chores can help make the most of your time and alleviate frustration. However, excessive daytime tiredness is not normal and should not be accepted as such. See your doctor if you feel excessive daytime fatigue.

BELOW **As life changes so do sleep patterns, therefore a sleep re-evaluation may be in order.**

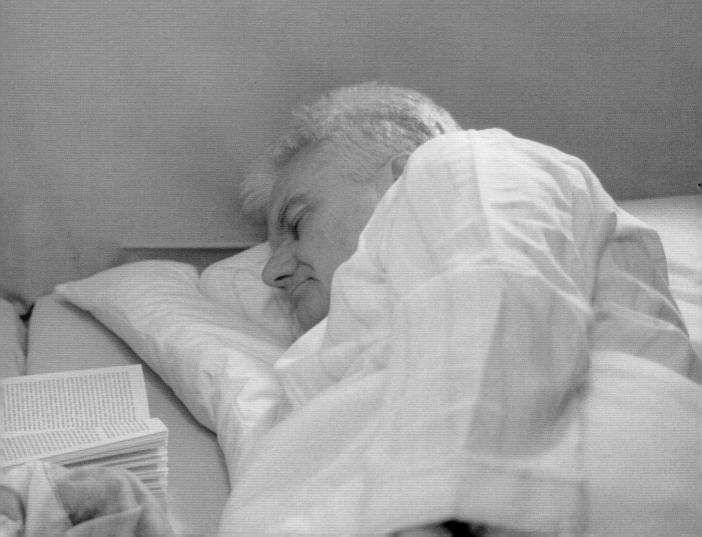

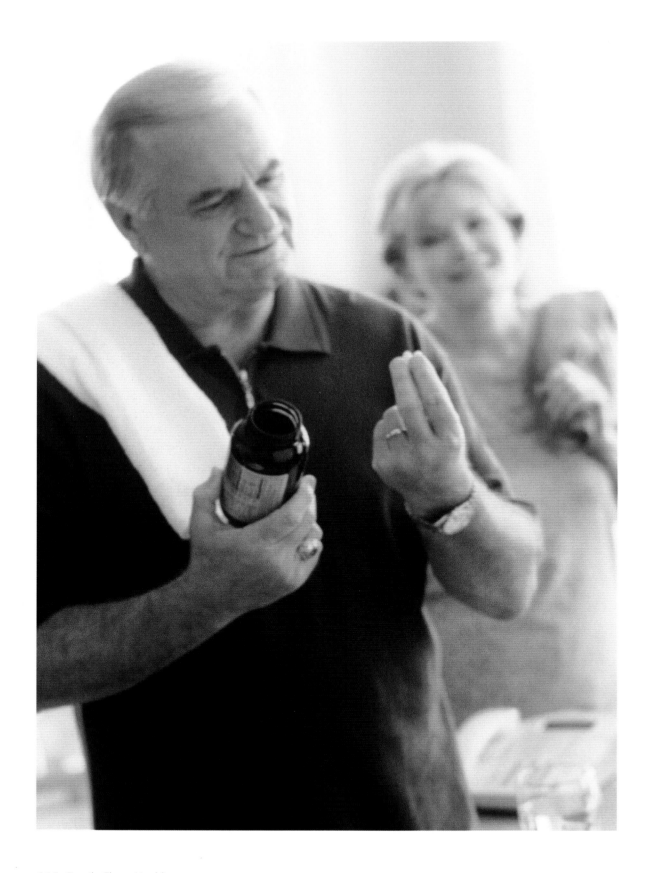

OLD AGE

As we know, babies spend at least 50 per cent in REM sleep, normal adults 25 per cent and in this later stage of life, this figure drops to only 15 to 20 per cent in the dreaming state. Older people also need less sleep, which is though to be linked to the drop-off in production of the growth hormone, and in the production of melatonin as we age. The amount of stage four (see also pages 12–14), deep refreshing sleep, is also reduced drastically. Most of our sleep in later years is made up of stage one and two non-REM sleep, which can also lead to more night-time awakenings, as in these stages we are more sensitive to noises that may jolt us.

Despite less REM sleep, senior citizens are much more likely to remember their dreams as they waken more often in the night. Sleep scientist Paul Martin suggests that as we enter old age, we lose roughly half an hour of night-time sleep every ten years. A study performed by Americas Stanford University found that of a sample of adults from 65 to 88, 40 per cent suffered from 'micro-arousals', awakenings lasting seconds, between 200 to 1,000 times a night. This was shown to have a direct relationship to daytime sleepiness. A short afternoon nap, however, has been shown to greatly improve alertness and mental performance; although you should experiment with naps to see what works. A short nap during the early afternoon works best; however avoid napping altogether for a while to see the naps could be the cause of poor night-time sleep.

Medication for various illnesses associated with ageing can often cause insomnia as a side effect, so speaking to a doctor should be the first step, in case a simple change in prescription can help. A doctor may also choose to prescribe a short-acting sleeping tablet that will not result in drowsiness during the day. Lavender has been shown to have exceptional results for helping the elderly overcome sleeplessness, and can be applied in drops on a pillow. Other age-related sleep difficulties are restless leg syndrome, sleep apnoea, and periodic limb movement, disturbing for a sufferer and their partner, all of which can be treated if diagnosed (see pages 28–31).

Taking control

Do a lifestyle stock take: review coffee, alcohol and nicotine intake as they can all be much more stimulating to an older person than to someone in their twenties. Stick to a rigid waking time, even if you have had a difficult night, and include some exercise early in the day, which will improve your mood, rest and general heath. A partner's illness may have made them a cause of disruption, or a beloved pet could be mouse-chasing in the middle of the night causing awakenings. Make sure your room temperature is correct; we become more sensitive to temperature as we sleep. Ask yourself if anything has changed recently that could be a cause. A 2003 poll carried out by the American National Sleep Foundation found a direct link between good sleep and a positive outlook and life experience in the elderly, and that those lacking in vital rest often suffered from undiagnosed sleep problems. Getting help could transform the quality of your waking hours as well as your slumber.

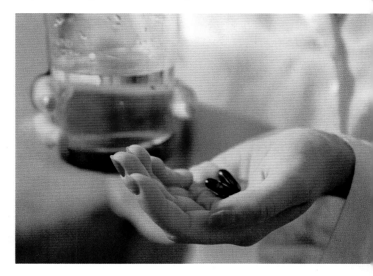

LEFT AND RIGHT **Medication can aid or disturb sleep; make sure you understand the effects of any prescribed.**

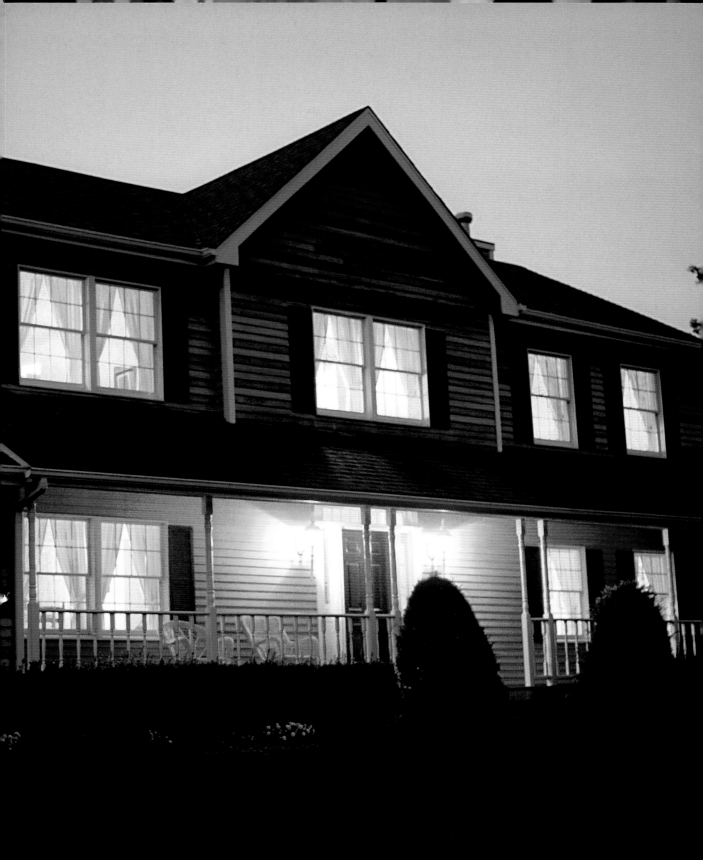

8 Sleep-Aid Programmes

Although the causes of insomnia and sleep-related problems are varied, there are several common methods to getting your sleep back on track. Here you will find three suggested programmes – one addressing stress and anxiety caused by daytime events, one for relieving persistent night-time wakenings, and one for a weekend catch-up to help put your sleep routine back on track.

You may prefer to devise your own tailor-made pre-sleep regime that includes writing in a journal or performing yoga, breathing or meditation exercises (see pages 80–4). Music is a great relaxer and can be used to supplement meditation and relaxation techniques; try nature sounds, mood music or light classical or jazz, but avoid anything with lyrics or spoken words or that is too loud or disharmonic, which will only serve to keep your mind stimulated.

TOUGH-DAY SLEEPLESSNESS SOLUTION

Some days we all find ourselves at home with a racing mind and an anxious to-do list, with a much-needed restorative slumber an impossibility. This usually means we find ourselves lying awake in the dark, trapped in a cycle of worrying about our inability to sleep. Try this relaxing 90-minute

LEFT **A retreat at the end of a busy day is essential for renewing your spirit and your body for the next day's challenges.**

programme to speed the onset of sleep, leaving you refreshed and able to start the next day energized and with a rebalanced outlook.

Step One

At the end of your active day, turn off your phone and switch on low lights around your home, including the bathroom (hard, overhead task lighting will not allow you to relax). Let your body adjust to the new lighting, encouraging melatonin production, and play soothing music. Especially useful are CDs specifically created for inducing sleep or deep relaxation. Have a warm bath and add five drops of mandarin or lavender essential to the water (see pages 73–9 for other excellent options). Leave the doors and windows closed to allow the atmosphere to become fragrant and steamy. Place a soft towel and bathrobe over a radiator to warm, and place a pen and note pad by the tub. While the bath is running, prepare and enjoy a soothing bromine- and tryptophan-rich snack, such as a wholemeal sandwich of banana and peanut butter, or turkey and lettuce with a glass of warm milk and honey. (See pages 50–3 for other foods that aid rest.)

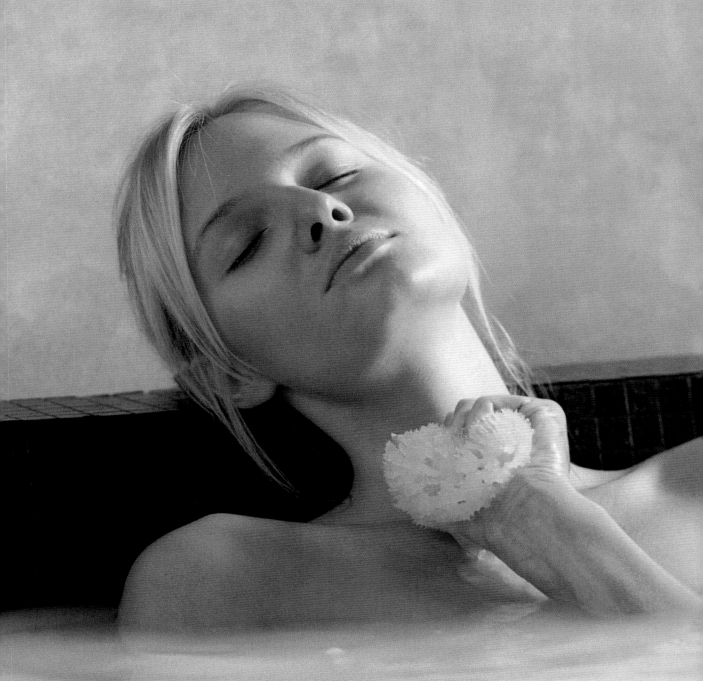

Step Two

Return to the bathroom where you need to soak for at least 30 minutes to allow the relaxing essential oils to work on your system. In the first few minutes in the tub, use the pen and paper to draw a list with three columns; tomorrow, one week, one month. When we are stressed, we see every problem as part of one big 'emergency' and writing each task under the relevant time frame will help you see what you really have to deal with. Once you have written out your tasks, ring each one that you can delegate or ask for help with (can you have your shopping delivered or ask a colleague to help source information for a report?). Write out your *real* to do list for the morning and put it to one side. Enjoy the remaining time in the water. After

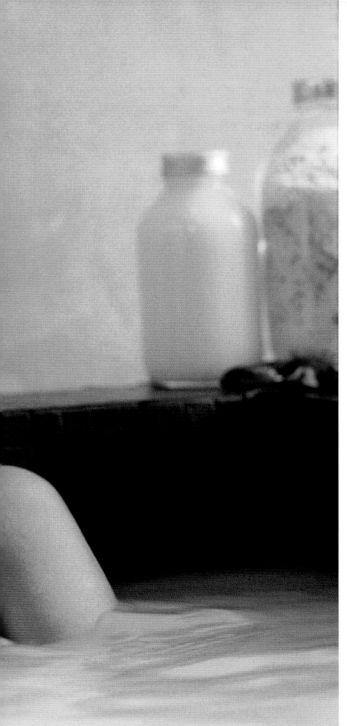

LEFT **When you take a relaxing bath, ensure that you allow at least 30 minutes for the essential oils to work their magic.**

Sit upright in a firm and comfortable chair. Begin to breathe in a slow, regular way (see also pages 82–3 on developing breathing techniques). concentrating on the inhale and exhale sensation. Now think of two words, such as 'calm' and 'relax', which equate 'rest' to you. When you breathe in, say one word in your mind, and as you expel the air, think of the other. Repeat for 5 to10 minutes. The technique will help banish other, worrisome thoughts that are hard to release with conscious effort. The more you practise and run through these steps, the more readily your body will respond; you are creating your own relaxation 'trigger'.

Step Four

Move to your bedroom and get into bed. Lie on your back in the Corpse position (see page 84) and begin some positive visualization to calm a racing heart and mind. Imagine a scene dear to you in which you were completely relaxed, perhaps on a winter holiday in a rustic ski chalet, lying on an old couch. Imagine the smell of the burning wood on the fire, then the sensation of the threadbare couch fabric, comfy underneath you. Then imagine the drowsy heat from the fire. Focus on different details and sensations in the scene, feeling yourself gradually relax. It may be that your ideal scene draws on a memory such as a picnic or a beach outing – just choose somewhere that you felt safe, happy and rested. This visualization technique should lull you off to sleep.

As another aid, create an 'emergency relaxation kit' consisting of a notepad, pen, essential oils or fragrant candles, self-massage tools and a music CD, which you can pull out after a harassed day for 30 minutes of instant relief. Make sure you maintain it so you don't find yourself turning the house upside-down for missing components, further adding to your stress.

your bath, dress in comfortable, loose sleepwear that makes you feel relaxed.

Step Three

Your body and mind need 30 to 60 minutes to wind down. Go to a comfortable, warm room and, in low light, try the following breathing method to help the body and mind release tension and worry.

NIGHT-TIME AWAKENING PROGRAMME

Night-time awakenings can be very distressing and isolating. It is essential to create a system to help manage these jolts, as they can rapidly become a source of great discomfort resulting in excessive daytime sleepiness. The first thing to appreciate is that everyone has night-time awakenings, several times a night, but usually they are so brief we have no recollection of them.

Step One

First, make sure you go to bed when you are sleepy; we often force ourselves to bed feeling tired, but the fatigued body is kept awake by a mind racing with dramas we have just seen on TV, in a brightly lit environment, not allowing the ourselves the preparation for sleep. Avoid daytime naps no matter how tempting if you are having this problem, to ensure you are truly tired. Some night-time awakenings can be caused by hunger and can be easily resolved; try a small tryptophan-rich meal 30 minutes before bed. It should be easy to digest, such as a glass of warm milk with nutmeg and honey.

Step Two

Some people wake with a jolt of panic or fear, a sudden adrenalin rush that pulls them into consciousness. The relaxation technique here was devised by Michael Krugman, founder of the Sounder Sleep System. After years of studying arts such as yoga, qigong and meditation, Krugman devised a system called 'mini moves™', which is based on breathing and visualization techniques and which helps achieve a state of deep relaxation and deep sleep. This adaptation is ideal for returning to sleep after a late night awakening.

1 Lie on your back in bed in a comfortable position, with a pillow under your head. Become aware of your breathing; is it anxious and laboured or are you feeling calm? Krugman calls this 'breath surfing'. Keep concentrating on your breathing until you feel completely focused on the sensation.

2 Move into the 'home position' by bending your arms at the elbows, still allowing the upper arm to rest comfortably by your side, and then place your hands – palms open, fingers slightly apart, thumbs wherever comfortable – on your chest, on either side of your sternum, tips of the fingers resting on the sternum. Everything should feel comfortable and loose.

3 Observe the movements of your breath, the rise and fall of your chest, feeling through your fingers.

4 Tune into the area underneath your thumbs. Slowly, begin to lift your thumbs a tiny way from your chest as your chest rises to inhale. Lower them as you exhale.

5 Synchronize your breathing and thumbs so each lift and breath corresponds in duration.

6 Stop, rest and feel. The anxiety should be gone, and your breathing fuller. Krugman says this practice will 'stimulate your body-mind's ability to sleep'. You may drift in a dreamlike state before nodding off.

Step Three

If you are still unable to return to sleep, get up, tidy the sheets and move to another room. You must avoid stimulating activities such as work and watching TV. Reading by lamplight, so that your body still appreciates that it is night, can soothe the mind, but avoid murder mysteries or anything overstimulating. Repetitive tasks such as ironing can help lull the mind back to sleep, or looking at a photography book such as rural landscape scenes with quiet music or nature sounds in the background can help. When you feel drowsy, and not before, return to bed. Repeat the 'mini moves'. Your body must associate only sleep with the bedroom. Avoid looking at a clock, but if you are still awake after 20 minutes, get up again and repeat.

Step Four

Despite a difficult night, get up at the same time. A regular wake time is essential for good rest, and trains the body to return to its natural pattern.

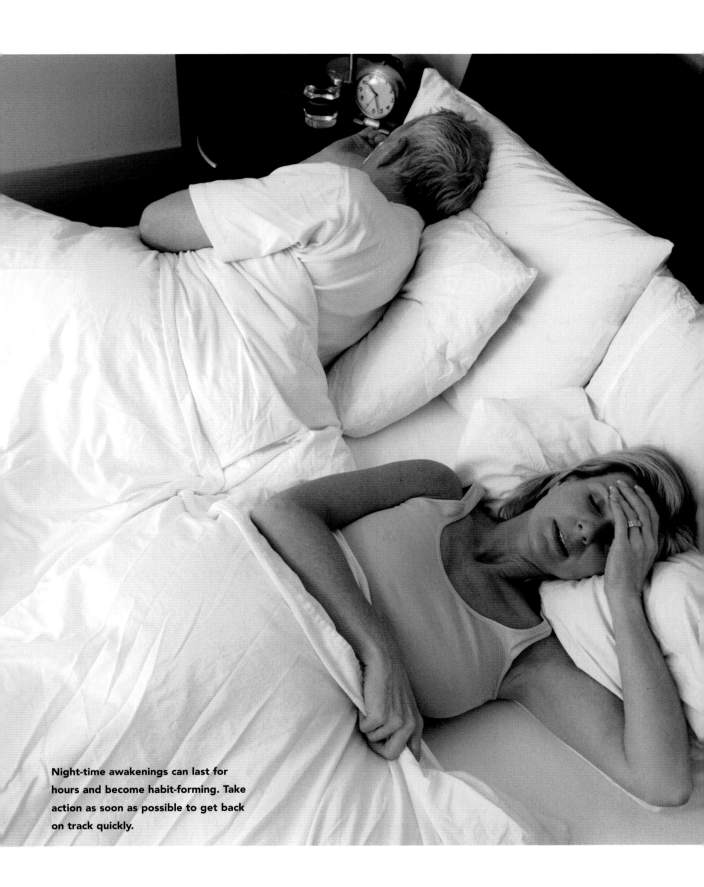

Night-time awakenings can last for hours and become habit-forming. Take action as soon as possible to get back on track quickly.

REJUVENATING WEEKEND REST PROGRAMME

As a matter of mental, physical and emotional health, we should all try to set a day a month aside to catch up on our sleep and neglected needs. This plan will help you enjoy a calm, relaxed day to help you unwind and attain a rejuvenating night's sleep.

Step One: Preparation

Choose a day when you don't work. Make sure to stock up on the recommended foods beforehand to prevent you from grabbing sugar-packed fuel, which will give you energy and mood spikes, and also eliminate the need to enter a busy and stressful supermarket on your 'recharge' day. Let friends and family know you are not available, unplugging the phone and leaving your computer and emails safely switched off. Try taking some gentle exercise such as a long walk or swim, as exercise is shown to improve sleep quality, but make sure you do this in the earlier part of the day (too near bedtime and you become overstimulated and unable to rest). Try booking a treat such as a massage or facial. If you are excessively tired, you may find yourself low at mid afternoon during your daytime circadian dip. Do something enjoyable that you rarely have the chance to do, like watch an old black-and-white movie, but try to avoid napping. This is a day of reward and nourishment, so a glass of wine with dinner is fine, but limit it to that; more will destroy sleep quality, as will stimulants such as cigarettes and caffeine. Keep yourself hydrated by drinking at least 2 litres (3½ pints) of water throughout the day.

Step Two: Diet

Choose food that will keep energy levels balanced all through the day, which will help you feel at peace and reduce the risk of an afternoon nap, keeping you awake later.

BREAKFAST

Choose slow-release carbohydrates such as an egg on brown or wholemeal toast or porridge. Try to

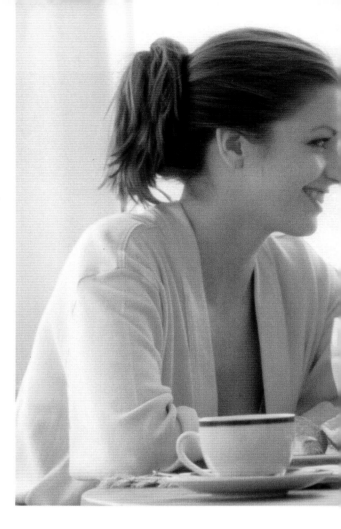

avoid caffeine, but if you feel unable to start your day without it make this your one cup, in order for it to leave your system by mid afternoon. Change to camomile tea throughout the rest of the day.

LUNCH

Include lean protein, such as fish, poultry or red meat, or soya, and green leafy vegetables; this will deliver a boost of vitamin B, great for combating the effects of a stressful week.

DINNER

This should occur at least two hours before bed and include carbohydrates such as brown pasta, rice or potatoes, pasta and lean protein, with a salad packed with healing antioxidants. A glass of mandarin or orange juice, which contains bromine, can also act as a sedative. Avoid spicy foods or excess sugar.

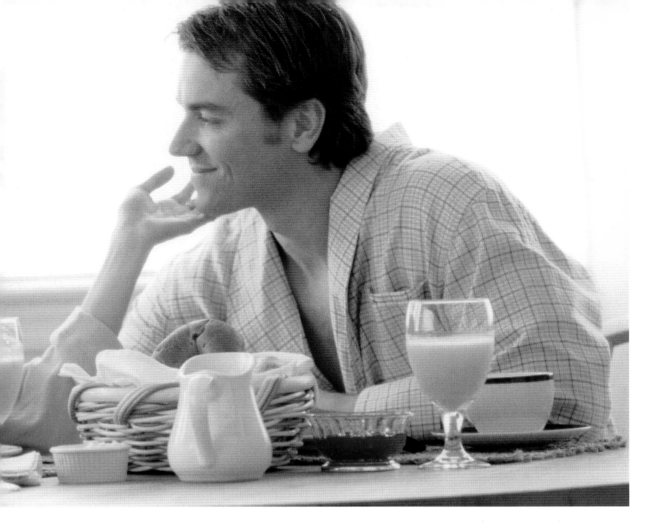

Step Three: Bathtime

Before bed, dissolve two cups of Epsom salts in a warm bath. The salts will help rid you of any of the toxins accumulated from previously eating and drinking excessively, and also relax the muscles. The salts can, however, leave the skin dry, so do moisturize well after your bath. You may like to add a few drops of bath oil to counteract the dehydrating effects of the salt. Those with skin complaints or high blood pressure should check with their doctor first. After your soak, dress in loose, comfortable nightwear.

Step Four: Massage

Move to your bed or a comfortable chair, using only a low light source and try this self-massage technique for releasing tension from your head, neck and shoulders. The scalp especially can hold a great deal of tension. Think of the sensation in

ABOVE **Choose a breakfast that offers slow-release energy to give you an energetic and positive start to the day.**

the forehead, when furrowing the brow or raising the eyebrows, which we often do when stressed.

Place the three middle fingers of each hand at the front centre of your hairline. Making firm circular movements, move in a straight line along the scalp down the back of your head to the hairline at the back. Move back towards the front, working your way gradually outwards until your whole scalp has been manipulated. End the massage by kneading the whole scalp rhythmically and softly.

Enjoy a relaxing read or listen to peaceful music, and when you feel tired, make your way to bed. Have a restful sleep that will help prepare you for the week ahead.

Keeping a Sleep Journal

K EEPING A DAILY JOURNAL documenting your sleep and lifestyle habits will help you understand your triggers for poor sleep and identify patterns that stand between you and getting a good night's rest. Answer the questions for the morning chart directly after waking up, and fill in the evening chart before you go to sleep. Getting enough sleep allows you to fight off disease, feel refreshed and able to function well during the day, and helps your powers of concentration and memory. If you continue to have trouble sleeping, take the record of your journal to your doctor for advice.

WEEKLY SLEEP JOURNAL: MORNING

	Day 1	Day 2	Day 3	Day 4	Day 5	Day 6	Day 7
What time did you first go to bed last night?							
How long did it take you to fall asleep?							
How many times did you wake during the night?							
How many hours did you sleep?							
At what time did you wake up?							
How did you feel when you woke up? (a) refreshed (b) neutral (c) tired							

WEEKLY SLEEP JOURNAL: EVENING

	Day 1	Day 2	Day 3	Day 4	Day 5	Day 6	Day 7
Did you nap during the day, and how much?							
Did you consume any coffee or alcohol? How much and when?							
How would you rate your daytime function? (a) energetic (b) somewhat energetic (c) neutral (d) somewhat tired (e) lethargic							

NOTES

RECOMMENDED READING

Caldwell, Paul J., *Sleep: The Complete Guide to Sleep Disorders and A Better Night's Sleep*, Firefly, 2003.

Choudry, Bikram with Bonnie Jones Reynolds, *Bikram's Beginning Yoga Class*, Thorsons, 2003.

Clarke, Jane, *Jane Clarke's Body Foods Cookbook*, Cassell, 2000.

Dement, William, *The Promise of Sleep*, Pan, 2001.

Hillard, Elizabeth, *Brilliant Colour at Home*, Kyle Cathie, 1999.

Holford, Patrick, *Patrick Holford's New Optimum Nutrition Bible*, Piatkus, 2004.

Kryger, Meir H., Thomas Roth Thomas and William C. Dement, *Principles and Practice of Sleep Medicine*, W.B Saunders Company, 1989.

MacEoin, Beth, *The Total De-Stress Plan*, Carlton, 2002.

Martin, Paul, *Counting Sheep*, Harper Collins , 2002.

Ryman, Daniel, *Aromatherapy Bible*, Piatkus, 2002.

Williams, Tom, *Chinese Medicine: A Comprehensive Guide for Health and Fitness*, Element, 1996.

RESOURCES

United Kingdom

Awake Ltd
67–69 Whitfield Street
London W1P 5RL
TEL: 0207 462 7660
EMAIL: info@awakeltd.info
WEBSITE: www.awakeltd.info

Allergy UK
Deepdene House
30 Bellegrove Road
Welling, Kent DA16 3PY
ALLERGY HELPLINE: 0208 303 8583
CHEMICAL SENSITIVITY HELPLINE:
0208 303 8525
EMAIL: info@allergyuk.org
WEBSITE: www.allergyuk.org

Association of Reflexologists,
27 Old Gloucester Street
London WC1N 3XX
TEL: 0870 567 3320
EMAIL: info@aor.org.uk

BackCare
16 Elmtree Road
Teddington, Middlesex TW11 8ST
TEL: 0208 977 5474
EMAIL: website@backcare.org.uk
WEBSITE: www.backpain.org

British Acupuncture Council
63 Jeddo Road
London W12 9HQ
TEL: 0208 735 0400
WEBSITE: www.acupuncture.org.uk

British Complementary Medicine Association (BCMA)
PO Box 5122
Bournemouth, BH8 0WG
TEL: 0845 345 5977

British Sleep Society
PO Box 247
Colne, Huntingdon
Peterborough PE28 3UZ
EMAIL: enquiries@sleeping.org.uk
WEBSITE: www.sleeping.org.uk

British Snoring and Sleep Apnoea Association
2nd Floor Suite, 52 Albert Road
North Reigate, Surrey RH2 9EL
TEL: 0173 724 5638
EMAIL: info@britishsnoring.co.uk
WEBSITE: www.britishsnoring.co.uk

The British Wheel of Yoga
25 Jermyn Street
Sleaford, Lincolnshire NG34 7RU
TEL: 0152 930 6851
EMAIL: office@bwy.org.uk
WEBSITE: www.bwy.org.uk

Cry-sis
HELPLINE: 020 7404 5011
EMAIL: info@cry-sis.org.uk
WEBSITE: www.cry-sis.org.uk
Support for families with excessively crying, sleepless and demanding babies.

Depression Alliance
212 Spitfire Studios
63–71 Collier Street
London N1 9BE
TEL: 0845 123 23 20
WEBSITE: www.depressionalliance. org

EHPA (European Herbal Practitioners Assoctiation)
8 Lion Yard, Tremadoc Road
London SW4 7NQ
TEL: 0207 627 2680
EMAIL: info@euroherb.com
WEBSITE: www.users.globalnet.co.uk/ ~ehpa/

Insomnia Helpline
TEL: 0208 994 9874
Trained nurses who will talk through problems and refer you to the right source for further help.

Loughborough Sleep Research Centre, Loughborough University
TEL: 0150 922 3091
EMAIL: Sleep.Research@lboro.ac.uk
WEBSITE: www.lboro.ac.uk/ departments/hu/groups/sleep/

Millpond Children's Sleep Clinic
TEL: 0208 444 0040
EMAIL: enquiries@mill-pond.co.uk
WEBSITE: www.mill-pond.co.uk/
client.html

Narcolepsy Association
Craven House, 121 Kingsway
London WC2B 6PA
TEL: 0845 4500 394
EMAIL: info@narcolepsy.org.uk
WEBSITE: www.narcolepsy.org.uk

**National Asthma
Campaign, (NAC)**
Providence House
Providence Place
London N1 0NT
TEL: 0207 226 2260
HELPLINE: 0845 701 0203
WEBSITE: www.asthma.org.uk

**Osteopathic Information Service,
General Osteopathic Council**
Osteopathy House
176 Tower Bridge Road
London SE1 3LU
TEL: 0207 357 6655
EMAIL: info@osteopathy.org.uk
WEBSITE: www.osteopathy.org.uk

**The Register of Chinese
Herbal Medicine**
PO Box 400
Wembley, Middlesex HA9 9NZ
TEL: 020 8904 1357

The Royal College of Psychiatrists
17 Belgrave Street
London SW1 8PG
TEL: 0207 235 2351
EMAIL: rcpsych@rcpsych.ac.uk
WEBSITE: www.rcpsych.ac.uk

The Shiatsu Society
Eastlands Court
St Peters Road
Rugby, Warwickshire CV21 3QP
TEL: 0845 130 4560
EMAIL: admin@shiatsu.org
WEBSITE: www.shiatsu.org

Sleep Apnoea Trust
7 Bailey Close
High Wycombe
Buckinghamshire HP13 6QA
TEL: 0149 452 7772
WEBSITE: www.sleep-apnoea-trust.org

**Sleep Assessment and
Advisory Centre**
10 Harley Street
London W1G 9PF
TEL: 0845 130 0933
WEBSITE: www.neuronic.com

The Sleep Council
WEBSITE: www.sleepcouncil.com

Sleep Studies Department
The London Clinic
20 Devonshire Place
London W1G 6BW
TEL: 0207 935 4444
EMAIL: info@thelondonclinic.co.uk
WEBSITE: http://www.lonclin.co.uk/

The Society of Homeopaths
11 Brookfield, Duncan Close
Moulton Park
Northampton NN3 6WL
TEL: 0845 450 6611
WEBSITE: www.homeopathy-soh.org

Surrey Sleep Research Centre
HPRU Medical Research Centre
Egerton Road
Guildford, Surrey GU2 7XP
TEL: 01483 682502
EMAIL: sleep@surrey.ac.uk
WEBSITE: www.surrey.ac.uk

North America
Better Sleep Council, Canada
PO Box 1277, Station B,
Downsview, Ontario M3H 5V6
WEBSITE: www.bettersleep.ca

Better Sleep Council, USA
501 Wythe Street
Alexandria, VA 22314–1917
WEBSITE: www.bettersleep.org

Canadian Sleep Society
080 Yonge Street, Suite 5055,
Toronto, Ontario M4N 3N1
TEL: (416) 483 6260
WEBSITE: www.css.to

**National Association for
Holistic Aromatherapy**
3327 West Indian Trail Road
PMB 144
Spokane, WA 99208
TEL: (509) 325 3419

**The National Sleep
Foundation (NSF)**
TEL: (202) 347 3471
EMAIL: nsf@sleepfoundation.org
WEBSITE: www.sleepfoundation.org

**Office of Dietary Supplements,
National Institute of Health**
6100 Executive Blvd,
Room 3B01, MSC 7517
Bethesda, MD 20892–7517
TEL: (301) 435 2920
WEBSITE: www.ods.od.nih.gov

**The Zero Balancing
Health Association**
Kings Contrivance Village Center
8640 Guilford Road, Suite 240
Columbia MD 21046
TEL: (410) 381 8956
EMAIL: zbaoffice@zerobalancing.com

Australia
**SomnoMed Australian
Sleep Association**
Principal Place of Business
Level 3, 20 Clarke Street
Crows Nest, NSW 2065
EMAIL: info@somnomed.com.au
WEBSITE: ww.somnomed.com.au

Australasian Sleep Association
GPO Box 295
Sydney, NSW 1043
TEL: 0500 500 701
EMAIL: sleepaus@ozemail.com.au
WEBSITE: www.sleepaus.on.net

INDEX

Figures in italics indicate captions.

5-HTP 112

acupressure 93, 117, 120
acupuncture 91, *91*, 93
adrenaline 38
Advanced Sleep Phase Syndrome 26
ageing 12, *16*, 17
aggression 23
alarm clocks 15, 31
alcohol 12, 24, 25, *25*, 26, 28, 31, 36, 39, 43, 47-8, *47*, 121, 122
allergies 62, *62*
alpha stage 20
alpha waves 12
alternative therapies 20
anxiety 7, 11, 32, *33*, 103-5
appetite 23
aromatherapy 74, *74*, 76, 93-7, 105, 107, 109, 111, 114, 117, 120, 122
asthma 25
Attention Deficit Hyperactivity Disorder (ADHD) 136
Awake 7

babies
birth of new baby 8, 11, 35, 40, *40*
sleep patterns 17, 125-9
teething 126
Bach flower essences 101, *101*, 105, 107, 109, 113, 122
bad breath 117-18
bathing 73-6, 87, 147-8
beauty sleep 8
bed 59-60
bedwetting 26, 136
behaving badly 24
bereavement 11, 35
beta waves 12
Better Sleep Council (US) 35, 36
body brushing 114
body clock 11, 26, *26*, 38, *122*
see also circadian rhythm
body temperature 23
brain power, boosting *19*
brain waves 12
breathing 23, 38, 82, 104
British Association of Counselling and Psyhotherapy 41
British Snoring and Sleep Apnoea Association 26
burn out 38

caffeine 31, 37, 43, 45, 105, 106, 110, 121
see also coffee; tea

calcium 54
Caldwell, Dr J Paul 36
Sleep Really Well 12
cancer 36
children
bedtime routine 134-5
pre-teens 136
chocolate 37
chromium 56-7, 109
Chronic Fatigue Syndrome 11
chronotherapy 26
circadian rhythm 11, *12*, 17, 26, 38, 47, 110
see also body clock
clutter 70, *70*, 73, 74
coffee 12, 28, 39, 43, *45*, 90, 105, 122
cold sores 119
colds 11, 118
colour 66, *66*, 68
Columbia University 7, 43
communication skills 23, 24
concentration 7, 50, 106-7, 110
confidence 24
continuous positive airway pressure (CPAP) device 31
cortisol 11, 38
co-sleeping 131

daytime sleepiness 110
death, premature 35
Deep Vein Thrombosis (DVT) 39
Delayed Sleep Phase Syndrome (DSPS) 12, 26
Dement, William 18, 125, 136
depression 7, 8, 25, 32, 36, 111-13
diabetes 7, 8
diet 20, 36, 43, 105, 106, 109, 110, 112, 114, 116-22
disasters, man-made 23
dreams *14*, 15, 17, 26
drinks
fizzy 43, *45*, 122
smoothie recipe 119
soothing *52*, *53*, 89
duvets 61

early rising, unwanted 17
EEG (electroencephalogram) 12, 15
electronic equipment 69, *69*
environment 116, 117
Epworth Scale 18
eucalyptus oil 28
evening primrose oil 57
exercise 7, 20, 36, 37, 39, 90, *90*, 114
eyes
bags under 8, 48, *48*, 121
dark circles around 120, 121
dry, itchy 23
eye pads 121
fatigue 7, 23, 114, *115*

Ferber, Richard 129
focus 106-7
foetus 125
folic acid 118
foods
aphrodisiac 87
energy-stabilizing 50-52
fatty 44
heavy, rich 43
processed 37
sedative 52
spicy 44

ginseng 57, 112
Glycaemic Index 50-51, *51*, 120
grief 25

Hamilton Anxiety Scale 32
headaches, recurrent 120
health 7, 8, *8*, 11, *14*, 89
heart disease 36
heart failure 31
herbal medicine, Western 99, 101, *101*
herbs 109, 117, 118, 120, 121, 122
holistic therapies 20, 88-101
homeopathy 98, *98*, 105, 107, 113, *113*, 114, 118, 120, 122
hormone production 11
hormone replacement therapy 140
humidifier 28
humidity 65
'hung over' feeling on wakening 117
hypersomnia 31

illness 11, 12, 25, 35
immune system 17, 36, 118
immunity, reduced 7
infections 8, 11, 17, 41, 118
inhibitions, loss of 24
insomnia 17, 20, *89*
causes of 25
chronic 25
extrinsic 25, 35-40
idiopathic 25
intermittent 25
intrinsic 25, 26-33
primary 24
psychophysiological 25
secondary 24-5
transient 25
iron supplements 31, 118
irritability 7, 23, 110

Jacobson, Dr Edmund 82
jet lag 12, 25, 36, 38-9, *38*, 122, *122*
Johns, Murray 18
K complexes 12
kava kava 57, 105
Krugman, Michael 150

'larks' 17, 26, 139, 142
lavender 145
libido 24, 116, *116*
lifestyle 7, 20, 28, 55
light therapy 26, 31
lighting 11, 64–5, *64*, 72, *72*
lips, chapped 23
lymph nodes 17

magnesium 31, 56, *56*, 118
Martin, Paul: *Counting Sheep* 18, 145
massage *20*, 76, 79, *79*, 93, 122
mattress 60, *60*
ME (Myalgic Encephalomyelitis) 11
medication 143, 145
medicine, traditional 20, 91, *91*
meditation 38, 80–81, *80*, 107
melatonin 11, 26, 36, 57, 74, *133*, 144
memory loss 7, 23
menopause 11, 35, 140, 143
menstrual cycle 140
middle age
    sleep patterns 142
minerals 54, 56–7
mood 7, *8*, 50, *50*, 109, *109*, 120
motivation 106–7
mouth guard 26, 28
music 72, *72*, 147

napping 18, 19, *19*, 36, 39, 110, 145
narcolepsy 25, 31, 110
newborns
    sleep plan 126
    trouble sleeping 126
nicotine 12, 47
    see also smoking
night-light 134
night terrors 26, 133
night-time awakenings 17, 26, 150–1
nightmares 26
nightwear 62
noise pollution 65
non-REM sleep 12, 15
norepinephrine 44
nutrition 7, 36
nuts 56

oestrogen 140
old age
    sleep patterns 145
Omega 3 oils 112
oral contraceptive pill 35
'owls' 17, 139, 142

pain sensitivity 23
paranoia 23
parasomnias 26
partner sleep 142

partying 12
periodic limb movement in sleep (PLMS) *15*, 31
phytonutrient herbs 109
pillows 61
polysomnography 28
Post-traumatic Stress Disorder 11
pregnancy 35, 140
premenstrual syndrome/tension 12, 140
progressive muscle relaxation (PMR) 8203

reflexology 93
reframing 104
relationships 8, *8*, 36, 84, *84*, 87, *87*
relaxation 38, 80–84, *104*
REM (Rapid Eye Movement) sleep 12, 15, 17, 35, 47, 61
resilience *19*, 23
respiratory failure 31
Restless Leg Syndrome (RSL) 20, 25, 31, 145
road accidents 7
Ryman, Daniele: *Aromatherapy Bible* 116

St Johns wort 112–13
salt 121
scent 72, *72*, *73*, 74, *74*, 76, 87, *87*
seasonal affective disorder (SAD) 31, *31*, 112
selenium 118
self massage *20*, 76, 79, *79*
sensory stimulation 69–72
serotonin 20
sheets 61, *61*
shiatsu 93, *93*
shift work 12, 17, 36
skin
    bad 23, 118–19, *119*
    puffy 120, *121*
    tone *48*
sleep apnoea 12, 25, 28, *28*, 31, 145
sleep clinics 31
sleep deficit 18
sleep diary 25, 90, *90*
Sleep Disorders Unit, Epworth Hospital, Melbourne 18
Sleep Latency Period 18, 110
sleep needs 18
sleep rituals 20, *20*, 73–9, 89, 147–53
sleep state misperception 25
sleep talking 26
sleep watches 15
sleepwalking 15
smoking 118, 121
    see also nicotine
snoring 12, 17, 26, 28, *28*, 140, 142
social skills 23

somnambulism 26
stages of sleep 12, 15
Stanford University, California 18
Stickgold, Robert 8
stimulants 12
stress 8, 20, *20*, 25, 35, 36–7, *37*, *38*, 41
sugar *48*, 49, 105, 106
supplements 54–7, 112, *112*, 114, 116, 118, 119, 120, 122
symptoms of sleep deprivation 8

task performance 8
teas 38, 39, 43, *45*, 89, 105, *112*, 122
teenagers
    sleep patterns 17
    sleep routine 139
    hormones 139
teeth grinding (bruxism) 26, 117
television 25, 59, 69, *69*, 134
temperature 65
texture 70, *70*
thyroid gland, overactive 11
toddler
    sleep patterns 129
tryptophan 51–2, *52*, 112
tyramine 44

virus infections 8, 11, 17
vision, impaired 23
visualisation 26, 38, *80*, 82, 83
vitamins 54
vitamin A 118, 120, 121
vitamin B complex 54, 105, 112, 122
vitamin B1 118, 121
vitamin B2 118, 121
vitamin B3 121
vitamin B6 118, 121
vitamin B12 118, 121
vitamin C 56, 112, 121
vitamin D 112
vitamin E 112

water, drinking 39, 45, *45*, 48, 121, 136
weekend rest programme 152–3
weight gain 7, 8, 12, 43
weight loss 28, 31
women
    hormones 140
work pressures 11, 25, 35
    see also shift work
work–life balance 35–6, *35*

yoga *20*, 83–4, *83*
corpse position 82, 84

zero-balancing 93
zinc 116, 118

PICTURE CREDITS

The publishers would like to thank the following sources for their kind permission to reproduce the pictures in this book.

Carlton Books Ltd: 57; Jason Bell: 119; Tom Leighton: 99, 62–63; Lizzie Orme: 56, 72, 75; Clare Park: 82, 83; Anna Stevenson: 20, 78; Polly Wreford: 42, 60, 61, 74, 76, 86, 94, 96, 97, 112, 120, 122; Mel Yates: 21, 58, 68, 71tl, 71tr, 71b, 87; Elizabeth Zeschin: 22, 67, 70

Corbis Images: Randy Faris: 135; Rob Lewine: 144, 152–153; Trinette Reed: 130–131; Larry Williams: 85

Getty Images: Botanica/Melanie Acevedo: 123; Gay Bumgarner: 30; Photonica: 1, 25, 92; Photonica/Erik Burass: 64; Photonica/David Clerihew: 66; Photonica Safia Fatimi: 106–107; Photonica/Issaque Fujita: 4–5; Photonica/Charles Gullung: 114; Photonica/Kazutomo Kawai: 53; Photonica/John Lamb: 110; Photonica/Clarissa Leahy: 41; Photonica/Jennifer Leigh Sauer: 91b; Photonica/Mecky: 142–143; Photonica/Takeshi Noquchi: 93; Photonica/Stephen H. Sheffield: 3, 15; Photonica/Daryl Soloman: 91t; Photonica/Mauro Speziale: 116; Photonica/Betsie Van Der Meer: 6, 9; Photonica/Craig Wetherby: 90; Photonica/Hiroshi Yagi: 26–27; Stephen Swintek: 37; Taxi/Tim Hall: 10; The Image Bank/Grant Faint: 24; Christopher Thomas: 54

Photolibrary.com: 17; Jessica Boone: 95; Bruce Byers: 146; Willard Clay: 100; Ichou: 80–81, 124; Macduff Everton: 115; Anthony Masterson: 138; Productions Digital: 145; Lisa Thompson: 73

Powerstock Zefa: AGE Fotostock: 39, 44, 48, 50, 111; AGE Fotostock/Liane Cary: 128–129; AGE Fotostock/Saxpix: 139; AGE Fotostock/Ben Walsh: 133

Rex Features: Phanie Agency: 127
ZEFA Picture Library, London: A.B./H. Winkler: 121; D. La Coppola/C. Meier: 16; S. De Geus: 51; Emely: 101; B. Erlinger: 13; Grace: 102, 104–105; A. Green: 40; Gulliver: 28–29; T. Hemmings: 141; U. Kaiser: 2; S. Krouglikoff: 148–149; LWA/Dann Tardif: 77, 137, 140; Linda: 34–35; /Masterfile: 151; Masterfile/Kevin Dodge: 134; Masterfile/Michael Goldman: 14, 18–19; Masterfile/Michael Mahovlich: 49; Masterfile/Matthew Wiley: 55; R. Morsch: 108–109; Newton: 46; Pinto: 88; E.Rian: 132; Sie Productions: 69; B. Sporrer: 113; Sucre Sale/E. Boivin: 45; Sucre Sale/P. Cabannes: 52; Turbo: 33

Every effort has been made to acknowledge correctly and contact the source and/or copyright holder of each picture, and Carlton Books Limited apologies for any unintentional errors of omissions which will be corrected in future editions of the book.